SOURCE BOOK

NATIONAL COMMISSION ON NURSING

An independent commission sponsored by
American Hospital Association, The Hospital Research and Educational Trust,
and American Hospital Supply Corporation

840 North Lake Shore Drive, Chicago, Illinois 60611

Written by Marjorie Beyers from issue papers presented by the commission, committee minutes, presentations to the commission, commission deliberations and data collected by the staff.

ISBN 0-87914-074-7

Trust Catalog Number: 654300

Printed in the U.S.A.

5M-12/83

CONTENTS

Acknowledgments

Throughout its three-year charter, the National Commission on Nursing collected data for this *Source Book* that comprised the information most pertinent to planning for the future. The publication represents the wide scope of input received by the commission from individuals, groups and organizations interested in nursing issues and problems and their resolution. This broad base of information reflects the commission's multidisciplinary membership: nurses, physicians, hospital trustees and chief executive officers, academicians and others. Input received from the commission membership's constituencies helped achieve a balanced view of nursing issues and future directions in health care.

Those who generously helped the commission can learn about the issues from the summary of information. The commission appreciates their help during the discovery and recommendation phases and hopes that this *Source Book* will be a useful adjunct to their future planning. The commission also appreciates the help of the Hospital Research and Educational Trust's communications department, James Boudreau and Lynn Bensen in preparing this publication. Many people now involved in projects and plans related to nursing can use the book in their planning. It is these people at local, state and national levels who are shaping nursing's future.

Preface

Current, up-to-date information is a valuable commodity for health professionals. Planning for the future requires data on which to base projections about trends and future events. This *Source Book* was developed in response to many requests for use of the commission's extensive data base for individual planning purposes.

Information selected for inclusion in this book was judged against three criteria. Information had to be:

- useful for policy development,
- generally applicable, and
- directed to understanding possible future trends in nursing.

Only the most pertinent information was selected for inclusion in the *Source Book.*

The publication includes overviews of the findings of the commission's public hearings, various invitational conferences and committee meetings and results of many of the commission's primary surveys. The *Source Book* not only provides information about data sources the commission used in developing its recommendations, but also can be used as a reference for those who are looking at the issues from their own perspective.

To increase its usefulness, the *Source Book* has been organized according to the chapters used in the commission's initial and summary reports. Together these chapters can be used for further study of the recommendations in the *Summary Report and Recommendations* or to explore possible action plans that may be developed from the data sources.

The *Source Book* is a tool that can be used for policy development and planning. It enables a long-range view of nursing issues and problems and it is a helpful resource for those who wish to quickly develop a perspective about future directions in nursing. New directions can be developed through thoughtful planning based on an understanding of the nursing profession today. In this regard, the *Source Book* is a tool for developing the future from the strengths of the present.

Marjorie Beyers, R.N., Ph.D.
Director
National Commission on Nursing

Chapter

1

INTRODUCTION

The *Source Book* is written to provide information relevant to:

- recruiting and retaining nurses in practice;
- enhancing job satisfaction;
- maintaining and increasing the competence and productivity of nurses in practice; and
- maintaining and improving the quality of nursing care.

These goals were established by the National Commission on Nursing in its work. The commission was an independent, multidisciplinary forum that brought together representatives from nursing, hospital administration, medicine, government, academia and business, hospital trustees and chief executive officers and others to deliberate about the issues and problems surrounding nursing. These issues needed to be clarified and placed in a historical context so that practical, long-range solutions could be developed. To be effective, solutions needed to involve the many disciplines associated with nursing.

It was agreed early on that a consensus in decision making was needed to make full use of the expertise and leadership of the commissioners. Consensus depended on open and honest sharing of views about the issues and deciding what could be done for future planning.

The commissioners recognized that their practical involvement in developing long-range solutions to nursing issues and problems had to be based on a common goal: to ensure high-quality, cost-effective patient care. Consensus in decision making among the many representatives on the commission was based on this common goal and the acknowledged interdependence of the members of this group to reach the goal.

To be effective, the commission needed to know the perceptions of people at the grass roots level. Therefore, the commission involved as many individuals, groups and organizations as possible in its activities to learn about nursing issues, problems and possible solutions. Many people and organizations provided testimony and information and responded to the commission's preliminary recommendations and documents. The interdependence of health professionals from many disciplines was evidenced in this input, as was the need for ongoing communication among key groups.

This publication begins by examining the trends the commission studied that affect nursing and society. It then considers nursing practice; credentialing, licensure and accreditation; and nursing education. A research piece on the environment and nursing practice discusses nurse job satisfaction and environmental effects on nursing. Supporting survey materials are included in the appendixes.

Insights gained from the many types of communication shared with the commission contributed to the strength of the commission's final recommendations. Some of the recommendations can be implemented immediately; others will take time to develop and put into action. It is action groups formed at local, state and regional levels and structured as representative bodies like the commission that will effect lasting changes.

Chapter

2

THE COMMISSION'S WORK

The National Commission on Nursing began its work in September 1980. It followed several sequential processes to reach its final conclusions about recommendations and action plans. These processes are described in this section.

Charge

One of the commission's initial actions was to approve the following charge to:

- analyze the internal and external forces that influence the environment of nurses at work;
- identify the effects of professional nursing and nursing-related problems on nursing practice in health care agencies;
- assess the professional characteristics of nurses in relation to the organizational structure of health care agencies;
- explore the motivation and incentives for nursing education and nursing practice;
- analyze the relationships among education, nursing practice and professional interaction in health care agencies;
- develop a platform of issues to be dealt with in the commission's activities; and
- plan methods to enhance the professional status and top management role of the nurse through:
  - — research to define status and role;
  - — publication of information to describe or explain the status and role in relation to health care; and
  - — demonstration projects to provide models for problem resolution, de-

velopment and reshaping relationships and structures in health care agencies.

To accomplish its charge, the commission confirmed its purpose to serve as a multidisciplinary forum that would deliberate on and develop action plans to resolve nursing issues and problems. In all of its work, the commission focused on factors that influenced the practice environment. The commission believed that defining nursing practice and educational requirements and establishing standards for nursing practice and credentialing were within nursing's purview. Practical goals the commission identified were: reduced turnover and attrition, improved cost-effectiveness and efficient nursing practice.

To help sort out the complex issues and problems surrounding nursing and to set a direction for deliberation and eventual recommendations, the commission needed a framework broad enough to encompass the many societal and institutional areas that influence nursing. This framework had to be specific enough to allow an in-depth study of the factors that most directly influence the environment in which nurses practice. Because of the complexity and interdependence of problems, the framework had to show how the context for the current nursing practice influenced the issues. It also had to illustrate the interrelationships between different issues.

Contextual and institutional factors that influence outcomes through interaction are shown in the framework illustrated in Figure 1. Contextual factors in society that most directly influenced nursing were perceptions, values and attitudes about the profession; economic factors; legal and regulatory practices; and interprofessional relationships in major institutions.

The major types of institutions related to nursing are educational and health care institutions, particularly hospitals. Within each type, variables that had a bearing on nursing were identified. The interface between these two major types of institutions was viewed as critical to achievement of nurse retention, job satisfaction and the effectiveness of nursing practice.

From the framework illustrated in Figure 1, the commission set forth criteria for selecting its activities and recommendations. Topics and activities the commission pursued were either:

- already fruitful or successful,
- in need of fresh approaches,
- amenable to demonstration,
- likely to generate the greatest impact, or
- short- or long-range and local, state, regional or national in scope.

The framework was further developed to define nursing's key relationships. The relationships between nursing and other disciplines were viewed as the medium for interaction within the total framework as well as for development of future improvements. Key relationships were divided into three broad areas:

- *Nursing Practice*, relations between nurses and:
  - patients;
  - physicians;
  - health care administrators and trustees;
  - health care institutions; and
  - the nursing profession;
- *Nursing Education*, relations between:

- the nursing profession and nursing education; and
- nursing education and nursing practice; and

- *Nursing and the Public.*

Figure 1

The national commission on nursing framework for deliberation, recommendations, action plans and research: identification of key relationships.

Contextual Factors	Institutional Factors	Outcomes
■ Economic ■ Societal ■ Status of women ■ Professionalization ■ Legal and regulatory ■ Interprofessional	Health care ■ Governance ■ Executive management ■ Interprofessional roles and relationships ■ Management: practices and policies • delivery systems • working environment • staffing • salaries • clinical ladders ■ Education: basic, graduate and continuing education ■ Transition from education to practice	■ Retention in practice ■ Job satisfaction ■ Practice performance ■ Efficiency and effectiveness of nursing care

Data Sources

After developing its framework, the commission conducted several activities to obtain data. In keeping with the spirit of openness that characterized the commission, many people were involved in the data collection. The commission sought information on how people felt about nursing issues and problems, what issues and problems were being dealt with at the grass roots level, what literature was available, and the outcome of nursing studies being conducted at state, regional and local levels.

Major sources of information came from public hearings and open forums; review of the literature, state studies and policy documents; responses to the *Initial Report and Preliminary Recommendations*, the *Survey of Innovative Programs and Projects* and other surveys; the National Invitational Leadership Conference; and the Invitational Conference for Nurses in Multihospital Systems. In addition, the commission made numerous site visits to hospitals and educational institutions with nursing programs; held conferences with individuals on specific topics such as the quality of nursing care measures; and received letters, documents and manuscripts from numerous individuals and organizations.

The Public Hearings

The commission knew that the issues and problems surrounding nursing had been examined in several major studies in many previous decades. What the commission needed to know was how the various groups involved viewed the issues and problems in 1980. To learn what people were thinking, the commission decided to hold a series of public hearings.

The commission requested and received testimony from nurses, physicians, hospital chief executive officers and trustees, public policymakers, researchers, consumers and others. Testimony also included studies from state, regional and local groups; public documents; issue papers; written testimony; and personal letters.

Public hearings held in six major cities in the United States provided many people with an opportunity to express their views about current issues and problems in nursing. The commission gained both perspectives and suggestions about how these people could work together to confront and resolve concerns.

In addition to the public hearings, the commission held three open forums in cooperation with the American Hospital Association's Center for Small or Rural Hospitals. At the open forums, the commission learned of the special problems and responses of the nation's 3,000 small or rural hospitals. Perceptions of nurses, hospital administrators and trustees from these hospitals were shared in both written and oral testimony at the forums.

Testimony received from the commission contained a wealth of information. Areas that needed further study were highlighted, solutions were presented, and the commission, putting all of the testimony from various groups together, obtained a more balanced perspective of the issues and problems.

The Literature Review

The commission's literature review was focused on factors that influence nursing practice. Topics for research in popular nursing literature included:

- the image of nursing,
- professionalization,
- nurse-physician relations,
- multidisciplinary health teams,
- nursing administration and governance,
- clinical ladders,
- nursing management and organizational issues,
- nursing education,
- educational mobility,
- transition,
- staff development programs, and
- continuing education.

The findings of the literature review were remarkably similar to issues and problems discovered from testimony at the public hearings.

State Studies and Policy Documents

State studies and policy documents were sent to the commission by various groups. Overall, the studies represented the work of state boards of higher education or the equivalent, state nurses' associations, state hospital associations and special projects involving one or more associations or multidisciplinary state or regional groups. Almost all of these studies contained data about a variety of issues including nurse supply, turnover and vacancy rates and often included recommended actions for meeting the demand for nurses.

Initial Report and Preliminary Recommendations

Deliberation about the nursing-related issues and problems continued as the commission progressed in its work. To let others know about its progress, the *Initial Report and Preliminary Recommendations* was published in 1981. This report contained the platform of issues and problems thus far identified by the commission and its initial recommendations for future actions.

The commission not only wanted to share its thinking, but it also asked for responses to the *Initial Report and Preliminary Recommendations* from the individuals, groups, institutions and organizations that would eventually take on the work of implementation. Each organization represented on the commission conducted a review of the *Initial Report and Preliminary Recommendations* by its membership. Processes for this review varied, but the resulting responses helped the commission complete its deliberations so that the outcomes would be useful and practical.

Surveys

The commission conducted several surveys in 1982 to learn more about selected aspects of nursing. More information about the purpose and use of these surveys is presented in the section of this *Source Book* to which they apply or in the appendixes.

A brief description of the *Survey of Innovative Programs and Projects* follows. The reader is referred to the publication of survey results for more information.

Survey of Innovative Programs and Projects

Phone contacts were made with state nurses' associations, state hospital associations and constituent leagues for nursing early in the commission's work. During these contacts many staff members openly shared information about nursing issues and problems pertinent to their geographic areas. They also shared information about successful programs and projects taking place in their areas. To find out more about the number, location and nature of these innovations, the commission conducted a survey of innovative programs and projects. The state associations were asked to identify innovators and disseminate survey forms. Invitations to participate in the survey also were published by the organizations represented on the commission.

Responses to the survey demonstrated that many institutions had initiated programs and projects to improve the environment for nursing practice. The commission served as a clearinghouse for this information by publishing the results of the survey.

These survey results were used in the commission's general data base and provide a broad level of information. Many new projects received by the commission after publication are described in a supplement to the first publication. This activity helped bring people with similar interests and concerns into contact with one another. The report lists a brief description of the program or project and contact persons to assist those seeking ideas or specific information.

The National Invitational Leadership Conference

In March 1981, the commission conducted a National Invitational Leadership Conference attended by teams from hospitals recommended by state health-related organizations as effective and innovative. Thirty hospitals representing a wide range in types of organizational control, size and geographic locations were represented at this conference. Each hospital team consisted of a trustee, chief executive officer, top nursing administrator and physician. These leaders met in groups according to occupation and also in teams from hospitals categorized by size.

At the conference, participants shared ideas about how to improve organizational effectiveness. Relationships in organizations that affected nursing and the quality of patient care were discussed from the perspectives of governance, administration and management of nursing services. The different perspectives of each group were clarified as the various leaders shared their innovative practices. Features common to progressive hospitals were identified as were common problems and goals. Differences also were discussed.

Chapter

3

THE SOCIETAL CONTEXT

Trends and Influences

The commission explored projected trends that would affect nursing in the future. Many of the societal trends affecting nursing were also having an impact on other sectors of society: demographic trends; attitudes about work and leisure; new types of family structures; and new societal views about women's roles, health and health care. What was happening to the 1.7 million registered nurses in 1980 was typical of society as a whole. The effects of the trends were sufficient to cause some fundamental changes in the way people viewed their employment and the expectations they had of their employers. Therefore, the commission studied the societal context in which nursing takes place beginning with an examination of societal trends and then focusing on how these trends affect the health care delivery system.

Societal Trends in the 1980s

Each decade has unique characteristics. The decade of the 1980s began with an attitude of ferment, a sense of uncertainty, a desire to improve the standard of living in a period of economic turbulence, a need to reassess major organizations, a need for unification in common policy goals and leadership to deal effectively with shifting values and resource accessibility. A common theme in the literature of the early '80s was the need to improve the quality of life. Better use of increasingly scarce resources to attain improved quality in all aspects of life was a recurring theme. Improved education, improved worker performance and productivity and improved standards of living in personal and community life were goals often cited.

Futurists project that in the environment of the '80s, innovations will be fostered in all sectors of society. Innovators are looking at what now exists and are studying what to retain, what to change and how to realign elements. Within society there are those who wish to restore traditional values, those who wish to establish a new social order and those who would prefer to continue existing practices. The result of interaction among people with these varying views will be influenced by factors such as demographic changes, emerging relationships between work and leisure, the economic and political tenor of the nation and what people decide to do in their own institutions and communities. Each community or group will decide how it defines quality of life according to its collective attitudes and values.

Demography

In health care, as in other types of business and industry, both productivity and consumption are related to demography. Greater segments of the population are aging, which influences the work force and the types of consumer products people will want to use. The median age in 1970 was 28 years; it is expected to shift to 35 years by 2000. About 70 percent of the work force in the year 2000 is projected to be between the ages of 25 and 44. There will be more people in the over-65 age group and an even more rapid rise in the over-75 year population. Later retirement and economic need will keep more people actively employed after age 65.

At the beginning of 1980, 51 percent of all women aged 16 and over and half of the women (16.6 million) with children under 18 were employed. It was estimated that, on the average, one-fourth of the total family income was earned by women. The size of families is expected to decrease: by 1990, 45 percent of households are projected to be headed by single persons. Women are expected to continue working because of many factors, including increasing educational levels, the trend toward smaller families, public acceptance of women at work, the entry of women into professions and the benefits accrued from employment. An improved standard of living, increased purchasing power for families and the desire to maintain a standard of living have been identified as benefits of employment by women.

Work and Leisure

People who are satisfied with their work tend to perceive that their quality of life is good, and they tend to be more productive in their work. Job enrichment, job design and other similar topics are part of the management language that reflects and finds ways to promote employees' satisfaction with their work. Walton (1979) proposed a three-level concept of work improvement. The first level includes work design techniques, the second level consists of work culture ideals and the third level comprises the desired outcomes for business and employees. Simply stated, the techniques create the culture that influences the outcomes for both the organization and the employees. In Walton's model, reshaping the work culture resulted from improving workplace design, creating pay systems based on performance and skill levels, involving employees in budget planning and implementation and instituting self-supervision, work teams and employee education to broaden job skills. All of these factors contributed to achieving improved employee satisfaction and organizational productivity.

Individuals seeking an improved quality of life are looking for job enrichment and for self-actualization and personal enjoyment in leisure. They are interested in balancing various facets of life. Economic unrest, the search for new values in the face of changing life-styles, elements of distrust and speculation about traditional organizations and the acknowledged expansion of technology and innovation are influencing the choices people are making.

Changes in Service Industries

The introduction of technology that changes the roles and functions people perform in their work is having a significant impact on the service industries, which account for approximately two-thirds of the gross national product. According to Lovelock and Young (1979), involving consumers in performing services is now more possible because of technological advances that allow for changing service delivery procedures. Customers increasingly are performing some of the functions previously provided by service industries. The "do-it-yourself" approach to acquiring services can stretch consumer purchasing power and increase the availability of services. These new uses of technology, however, involve changing consumer habits and behaviors and teaching consumers to use services differently for their convenience and enjoyment. Computer-controlled gasoline service pumps, automated post office stations and other innovations are examples of how technology is enabling more flexible consumer participation in performing services.

Growth of Technology

Technology is purported to flourish in societies characterized by competition, adequate capital, energy and human resources; a flexible educational system geared to train, retrain or otherwise help people adapt to the new technology; and an acceptance that many skills may have a shortened lifespan. Technologic advances thus would be slowed by deficits of capital and energy resources; inability of educational systems to keep pace with innovation; slowness of organizations to accommodate changes; resistance to change within work structures, unions and among employees; and concern about the possible effects of technology.

Health Values

Health is a component of all facets of life. Changes in attitudes and values about health care appear to be occurring rapidly. Current development of coalitions for health involving community leaders, industry and business as well as health-related agencies and organizations demonstrate the rapid change in views about health. At an individual level people appear to be involved in activities to maintain their own health. At the same time, there are many current issues about accessibility to health care and how to use the technology of health care that raise moral and ethical issues.

Nurses perceive their roles and functions according to what is happening within the societal context. Peter Drucker has called the United States of the 1980s the "employee society." Institutions in this society are the source of livelihood, opportunity, status, function and personal fulfillment. As such, employers and employees have certain expectations of society's institutions. Nurses will be affected by changes in health care both as consumers of health care and in their role as clinical practitioners.

Though the commission focused on hospital nursing, nurses function in all other sectors of the health care system. Projections about health care delivery in the future will therefore affect nursing in all of its practice settings. To examine trends that would affect nursing most directly, four factors affecting the delivery of health care were isolated for review:

- the population to be served,
- health care services to be provided,
- resources needed to provide health care services, and
- the system for health care delivery.

The Population To Be Served

Health care needs of the population are influenced by age. Preventive health care predominates for people in the younger age groups; use of acute and chronic care services increases as age advances. Major shifts expected in numbers of people within different age groups will therefore influence services needed. Shifts expected for the next 30 years are:

- a gradual increase in the number of persons below the age of 25;
- a steady, sharp decrease in the number of persons aged 24 to 44;
- a slight decrease in the number of persons aged 45 to 64 until 1990, followed by a sharp increase to the year 2000, and then a slow decrease to the year 2010;
- a gradual decline in the number of persons aged 65 to 74 until the year 2000, followed by a sharp decrease thereafter; and
- an increase in the number of persons 75 years and older until 1990, followed by a steady decrease in this age group.

Health Care Services To Be Provided

Projected trends in health care use based on current patterns indicate that the major changes in use of services to 1990 will occur in age groups below 25 and over 75 years. The under-25 age group will use more preventive health care services and the over-75 age group will use more chronic and long-term health care services. Increases in population in both of these groups indicate increased use of preventive, chronic care and long-term services. Shifts in population occurring after 1990 are projected to change use of health care services again. An increased number of people between ages 45 and 64 and a sharp increase in the number of people between ages 65 and 74 indicate increased use of acute health care services by this over-45 age group. Increased use of chronic and long-term services are projected to increase as the population between ages 65 and 74 continues to increase.

Resources Needed to Provide Health Care Services

All categories of health care services—preventive, acute, rehabilitative, chronic and long-term—will continue to be needed by the population as a whole. Demographic changes indicate shifts in the level of use of each service category. If current trends continue, future health care services will be increasingly influenced by growth in technology and the economic situation. The projected increase in medical technology will not only change treatment for diseases, but also is expected to change the way services will be delivered and the resources needed to deliver them. A reduction in the rate of growth of health care spending is the overriding economic theme reflected in the literature.

Health Care Spending Influences

To examine the effects of reducing the rate of growth in health care spending, three main factors were examined: funding sources, major expenditures and the location of services. Relationships among these factors are expected to continue changing in the future. How they will change is uncertain.

Assumptions made about evolving trends were:

- There will be changes in the way health care is delivered as sources of funding continue to change. Overall, there will be a decreased rate of growth in health care spending;
- Manpower, including all types of health care professionals, will continue to be a major expenditure in health care services. The trend to employ fewer but more qualified health professionals will continue;
- Technologic development will continue with emphasis on less invasive and more efficient modes of diagnosis, treatment and patient care. In addition, technology will influence communications and operations management in and among health care institutions; and
- Education of health professionals will continue to be upgraded and related to current and future developments. Increased use of communications technology, selectivity of applicants and modes of continuing education that relate to expansion in knowledge are projected.

The System for Delivery of Health Services

Knowing that trends point toward change in the system for delivery of health care services and that the shape of future health care delivery is uncertain, the commission developed a model for ongoing evaluation of events. This model illustrates the relationships among funding sources, major resource expenditures and the location of services (Figure 2), and is useful for an ongoing examination of trends.

In the model, nursing as a clinical practice discipline would be most directly affected in the areas of major resource expenditures, including manpower, technology, education and research, because nursing is patient-care focused. Nursing's input into the system would be based on providing care most effectively and efficiently in the various locations of services: hospitals,

Figure 2

Model of relationships among funding sources, major expenditures, and location of services in the health care delivery system.

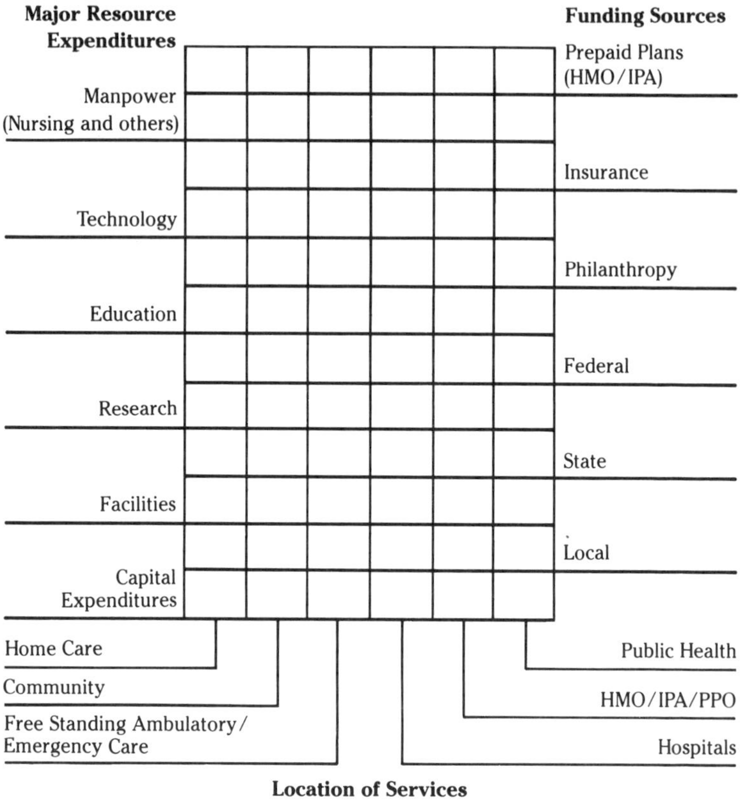

free-standing service centers, health maintenance organizations and other prepaid group plans, community and public health programs and long-term and extended home care services.

Threads of influential factors that flow through this model are technologic progress; the capability of all types of organizations, within health care to form new linkages and new structures in technologic processes and systems; and perhaps, the ingenuity of innovators in developing useful technologic applications for health care delivery. Increased use of technology implies the necessity of an educational system that is flexible enough to allow for retraining or other methods to help employees adapt their skills to new technology. It implies acceptance of a shorter life span for skills and a need for a broader knowledge base from which adaptations can be made.

Given the trends, relationships between nursing and health care organizations will probably change. Organizational structures and modes of nursing care delivery are changing toward models that promote better utilization of nursing knowledge, more efficient use of assisting personnel and increased participation of nurses in decision making that affects nursing practice. Other professional health disciplines are likely to be similarly affected by the trends noted in this section and the changes in organizational structures will involve changes in the interrelationships among the health care disciplines.

As these changes occur, conflict and accommodation are expected. There will be conflict and accommodation in evolving types of relationships between professionals and institutions. All of these changes will continue to be influenced by overall societal trends. Changes in health care delivery will continue to reflect prevailing societal attitudes and values. Goals to improve the performance and efficiency of employees and organizations and satisfaction of nurses are all predicated on the primary goal of delivering quality patient care.

Directions for Nursing

Nursing must take a giant step forward to be ready for the health care delivery system of the future. Methods that will transcend current issues and problems and move nursing forward are essential. Nurses capable of providing care in high-technologic, high-intensity patient care situations will be needed. In this regard, the following assumptions were made about the future directions for nursing in clinical practice settings:

- trustees and hospital or health care agency chief executive officers will increasingly control health care spending and will demand of physicians, nurses and other health professionals the mechanisms for selection and monitoring of health professionals' competency;
- administrators of health care agencies will play a central role in organization and management of the environment for care;
- physicians, nurses and other health professionals will increasingly participate in planning, policy development and executive management related to patient care;
- clinical practice of all types of health professionals will be supported by technology and efficient management systems;
- moral and ethical issues will have greater prominence in health care as technologic capabilities increase and costs are constrained; and
- more efforts will be directed to humane, compassionate care to counterbalance the effects of technology on patients.

Increasing demands will be placed on nursing to fulfill patient caring roles. There will be new equilibrium established as nurses and physicians, whose roles are similar, undergo conflict and competition, differentiate their roles and functions and increasingly cooperate in providing a total range of patient services.

Bibliography

Abel-Smith, B. *Sharing Health Care Costs.* DHEW Pub. No. (PHS) 79-3256. Washington, D.C.: Office of Health Research, Statistics and Technology, National Center for Health Services Research, 1980.

Abernethy, D.S. and Pearson, D.A. *Regulating Hospital Costs: The Development of Public Policy.* Ann Arbor: Alpha Press, 1979.

Ahearn, M.C. *Health Care in Rural America.* Washington, D.C.: U.S. Department of Agriculture, 1979.

____________. *Health: What They Know, What They Do, What They Want.* Survey conducted by The Innovative Group. LaJolla, CA: American Hospital Association, 1978.

Carter, L.J. and Spaeth, G. Planning for the 'consumer society.' *Science* 208:1009, May 1980.

Cetron, M. and O'Toole, T. Careers with a future: Where the jobs will be in the 1990s. *The Futurist* 16:11, June 1982.

Church, R.L. and Sedlak, M.W. *Education in the United States.* New York: The Free Press, 1976.

Cook, G. RX for the maladies of health care: A medical revolution in the making. *The Futurist* 13:179, June 1979.

Culleton, B.J. Health care economics: The high cost of getting well. In Abelson, P.H. (ed.), *Health Care Regulation, Economics, Ethics, Practice,* p. 41. Washington, D.C.: American Association for the Advancement of Science, 1978.

Donahue, T. and Oliva, N. M.A.S.H. moves to main street. *The Futurist* 16:20, Aug. 1982.

Drucker, P.F. The 're-industrialization' of America. *Wall Street Journal* LX:1, June 13, 1980.

Edmunds, S. Three economic scenarios for the '80s. *The Futurist* 14:12, Dec. 1980

Enthoven, A.C. The consumer choice approach to national health insurance: Equity, the marketplace, and the legitimacy of the decision-making process. *Effects of the Payment Mechanism on the Health Care Delivery System.* DHEW Pub. No. (PHS) 78-3227. Washington, D.C.: U.S. Government Printing Office, 1977.

Freeland, M., Calat, G. and Schendler, C.E. Projections of national health expenditures, 1980, 1985, 1990. *Health Care Financing Review* I:1, Winter 1980.

Fried, C. Equality and rights in medical care. In R. Munson, *Intervention and Reflection, Basic Issues in Medical Ethics,* pp. 450-56. Belmont, CA: Wadsworth Publishing Co., Inc., 1979.

The General Mills American Family Report, 1978-79: Family Health in an Era of Stress. Conducted by Yankelovich, Skelly and White, Inc. Minneapolis: General Mills, Inc., 1979.

Guzzardi Jr., W. Demography's good news for the eighties. *Fortune* 100:92, Nov. 5, 1979.

Hancock, T. Beyond health care. *The Futurist* 18:4, Aug. 1982.

Kane, R.L. and Kane, R.A. Care of the aged: Old problems in need of new solutions. In Abelson, P.H. (ed.), *Health Care Regulation, Economics, Ethics, Practices,* pp. 100-106. Washington, D.C.: American Association for the Advancement of Science, 1978.

Kouzes, J.M. and Mico, P.R. Domain theory: An introduction to organizational behavior in human service organizations. *Journal of Applied Behavioral Science* :449.

Lovelock, C.H. and Young, R.F. Look to consumers to increase productivity. *Harvard Business Review* 57:168, May-June, 1979.

Marland, S.P. Liberal education and work, united from the beginning and for all. In Solomon, L.C., *New Directions for Education and Work: Reassessing the Link Between Work and Education*, p. 39. San Francisco: Jossey-Bass, Inc., 1978.

Matek, S.J. *Accountability: Its Meaning and Its Relevance to the Health Care Field.* DHEW Pub. No. (HRA) 77-72. Washington, D.C.: U.S. Government Printing Office, 1977.

Mills, D.Q. Human resources in the 1980s. *Harvard Business Review* 57:154, July-Aug. 1979.

Morison, R.S. A further note on visions. *Daedalus* 109:55, Winter 1980.

Mosteller, F. The next 100 years of science. *Science* 209:21, July 4, 1980.

Mushlin, A. and Appel, G. *Developing a Quality Assurance Strategy for Primary Care.* National Center for Research Institute, 1980.

Myerhoff, B. Number our days. *Natural History* 88:77, Mar. 1979.

Office of Technology Assessment. *Assessing the Efficacy and Safety of Medical Technologies.* Washington, D.C.: U.S. Government Printing Office, 1978.

Plumleigh, G.E. Schools for the eighties: 27.5 miles per gallon. *Phi Delta Kappan* 61:24, Sept. 1979.

Saward, E. and Sorenson, A. The current emphasis on preventive medicine. In Abelson, P.H. (ed.), *Health Care Regulation, Economics, Ethics, Practice,* pp. 49-54. Washington, D.C.: American Association for the Advancement of Science, 1978.

Selim, R. Health in the future: In the pink or in the red? *The Futurist* 15:329, Oct. 1979.

Sheldon, A. and Barrett, D. The Janus principle. *Health Care Management Review* 2:77, Spring 1977.

Silberman, H.F. The relationship of education and work. In Solomon, L.C. *New Directions for Education and Work: Reassessing the Link Between Work and Education,* p. 21. San Francisco: Jossey-Bass, Inc., 1978.

Stander, I. The future of worker's compensation. *Medicolegal News* 8:7, Apr. 1980.

Stout D.K. The impact of technology on the economic growth of the 1980's. *Daedelus* 109:159, Winter 1980.

Survey conducted by Louis Harris and Associates, Inc. Pacific Mutual Life Insurance Company, 1978.

U.S. Department of Health, Education and Welfare. *The Impact of Health System Changes on States' Requirements for Registered Nurses in 1985.* DHEW Pub. No. (HRA) 79-8. Washington, D.C.: U.S. Government Printing Office, 1980.

____________. *Evaluation of Health Manpower Shortage Area Criteria, Bureau of Health Professions, Division of Health Professions Analysis.* DHEW Pub. No. (HRA) 80-20. Washington, D.C.: U.S. Government Printing Office, 1980.

Walton, R.E. Work innovations in the United States. *Harvard Business Review* 57:88, July-Aug. 1979.

Wirtz, W. Bridge building between education and employment. In Solomon, L.C. *New Directions for Education and Work: Reassessing the Link Between Work and Education,* p. 35. San Francisco: Jossey-Bass, Inc., 1978.

Wise, R.I. and Charner, I. Higher education and the labor market: Implications of new concepts for equity. In Solomon, L.C. *New Directions for Education and Work: Reassessing the Link Between Work and Education,* p. 11. San Francisco: Jossey-Bass, Inc., 1978.

Chapter

4

NURSING PRACTICE

Attitudes and values about nursing held by hospital trustees, health care administrators and others influence the nursing practice environment. These attitudes and values assume tangible form in the governance, administration and management structures of health care institutions and in critical working relationships between nurses and physicians.

Improving Relationships: Attitudes and Values

Improving relationships between nursing and other disciplines depends on the extent to which nursing is valued as a professional clinical practice. When nursing is valued as a professional clinical practice, the knowledge and skills of nurses are better utilized in quality patient care. Five major categories of issues abstracted from testimony at the commission's public hearings were:

- status and image of nursing, including changes in the nursing role in response to new variations in health care delivery and professional growth, as well as the corresponding changes in interprofessional relationships and public image;
- interface of nursing education and practice, including current and potential models for basic and graduate education and continuing nursing education to prepare nurses for practice and professional interaction in health care delivery;
- effective management of the nursing resource, including the mix of organizational factors required for nursing job satisfaction: staffing, scheduling, salary and benefits, support services, mode of care delivery, career development, manpower planning and recruitment and retention strategies;

- relationships among nursing, medical staff and hospital administration, including nurses' ability to participate through organizational structures in decision making as it relates to nursing care, the value and development of collegial relationships among health care professionals and the development and operation of interdisciplinary patient care teams; and
- maturing of nursing as a self-determining profession, including nursing's right and responsibility to define and determine the nature and scope of its practice, the need for and the role of nursing leadership, the potential of collective action to increase decision making in nursing practice and the need for unity in the nursing profession.

Each of these categories of issues is in itself complex. The complexity deepens when viewed from the different perspectives of the various individuals and groups seeking solutions.

Staff Nurses

Staff nurses viewed nursing's issues and problems in the context of caring for people and having sufficient authority and responsibility to make decisions necessary to fulfill their compassionate, supporting role in patient care. They saw themselves as both people in society and as employees of health care agencies and wanted to participate in decisions that affected them directly in patient care.

Nurse Administrators

Nurse administrators viewed the issues and problems from the perspective of developing nursing as integral to management and clinical decision making. At the same time, administrators sought to balance the need for ensuring nurses' caring role and function in providing quality nursing care with cost containment, demands of regulation and the best utilization of the nursing resource.

Hospital Administrators

Hospital administrators saw nursing care as essential to patient services. The nursing manpower issues and problems were seen as issues of maintaining quality patient care in the face of many other concerns about environmental pressures, new economic realities, cost containment and regulation that influenced the ability to maintain stable operations in the face of change.

Nurse Educators

Nurse educators viewed the issues and problems in relation to maintaining nursing as a legitimate professional clinical discipline competing for limited fiscal resources, qualified students and faculty and adequate patient care experiences for students.

Physicians

Concerned with medicine's emerging legal and professional issues and problems and the effects of new technology and changing relationships with health care agencies and funding sources, physicians wanted assurance that adequate numbers of qualified nurses would be available to care for patients.

State Planners

State planners viewed the confusion and lack of agreement about nursing as an impediment to rational planning for allocation of educational resources to ensure that enough nurses with the appropriate level of education would be available to care for patients in different practice sites.

Consumers

Confused about the many types of nursing education programs, consumers were seeking responsible and compassionate nursing care.

Trustees

Concerned with policy, long-range planning and resource allocation, trustees were seeking strategic plans that would ensure adequate numbers of qualified employees to provide quality patient care and fiscally responsible human resource management in health care settings.

Understanding Perspectives

Perspectives on the issues and problems held by different groups were affected by differing practice sites and regions of the country. Similarities across the United States were also apparent, as indicated by findings from the commission's National Invitational Leadership Conference (see *Nursing in Transition: Models for Successful Organizational Change*). Similarities in perspectives of hospital trustees, chief executive officers and nurse executives within the structures of hospital governance and administration were described. Based on the information gathered from the 30 hospitals represented at the conference and some site visits by the commission, models for these roles developed.

Governance

The relationship of the governing board to nursing was clarified. The board has the authority and responsibility for patient care and quality of services. It determines policy, external relationships and the hospital's mission, strategic plans, goals and objectives. The board develops resources and ensures appropriate maintenance and use of those resources. The board is responsible for development of human resources to ensure a quality staff for quality patient care.

Trustees indicated that it is appropriate to involve nursing in the policy development process within the institution. In a few of the represented hospitals, the top nurse administrator was a board member; in others, the nurse administrator was a member of board committees. In most of the represented hospitals, the nurse administrator had access to the board with responsibility to participate in planning and with reporting accountability. The critical element in nurse-board relationships was the board members' need to be provided with current information about nursing essential to meeting their responsibility for ensuring a quality nursing staff.

Hospital Chief Executive Officers

The hospital chief executive officer is responsible for the administration of the hospital and for external relationships. The CEO has a key role in ensuring an environment for quality nursing practice. The CEO's philosophy and the organizational structure were major influences on how nursing practice was recognized in the hospital, as well as on the quality of administrator-nurse-physician relationships. For example, they influenced:

- placement of the top nurse administrator in executive management;
- management and leadership skills of nurse managers and clinical specialists;
- competence of nurse credentials and educational programs; and
- the interdependent relationship of nursing to other departments—
  - — non-clinical (housekeeping, information systems, materials management), and
  - — clinical (pharmacy, therapies, diagnostic services).

Nursing represents the largest single professional group of employees in hospitals. Millions of dollars are allocated to nursing department budgets. To manage this vast resource, nursing administrators should have access to the board of trustees and participate in administrative committees and in policy and budget development. The top nurse administrators in hospitals following this structure are members of the executive management team. They participate with chief executive officers, other administrative level personnel and physicians in developing policies and plans to improve the quality of patient care.

Chief executive officers, however, are balancing environmental pressures and internal pressures. Nursing is one of many areas of responsibility. The transition of nursing to a clinical department was perceived by some to have the potential to disrupt relationships among employees in the entire institution. A delicate balance exists in many health care agencies among the different types of employees who are seeking relative status and recognition. The changes in nursing thus require revamping attitudes, enlightening colleagues and instituting administrative and medical staff recognition of nurses. To be effective, however, the top nurse administrator has to be qualified for the role.

The Nurse Administrator

The overall responsibility of the top nurse administrator is to create the environment for clinical nursing practice. Organizing nursing services, developing a leadership cadre of qualified nurse managers and clinical specialists and promoting cooperative relationships with administrators and physicians are elements of the nurse administrator's function. The nurse administrator has to establish and maintain nursing as a management unit defined as an organizational unit with its own hierarchy and subdivisions of responsibility. This management unit must allow authority and decision making by nurses in matters affecting the environment of practice and clinical patient care.

Effective participation of the top nurse administrator in executive decision making has many benefits. Nursing's input is helpful in organizational policy development and planning and also results in staff nurses feeling a stronger sense of belonging and organizational support for their efforts. In this type of environment, nurses felt that they had more decision-making authority and more organizational support to give high-quality nursing care.

Qualified Nurse Managers and Clinical Specialists

Having qualified nurses in managerial and leadership positions within the nursing department was essential to making appropriate decisions at the patient care level, as well as other management levels in the hospital. In regard to nursing practice, clinical specialists helped nurses upgrade their patient care knowledge and skills. They also cared for patients with complex problems. Increasing competence promoted recognition of nurses for their contribution to patient care; this recognition continued to stimulate an even better quality of patient care. Nurse-physician relationships were improved. Increased numbers of qualified, competent nurses changed the type of management and administration needed. Competent nurses required less supervision and oversight; more nurses were interested in developing their careers in an environment that was perceived as less bureaucratic. Thus, to accommodate the increased complexity of patient care, hospitals were upgrading nursing, reducing supervision and oversight and experiencing increased efficiency, increased retention and increased quality of patient care.

Nursing Department Organizational Structures

The nursing department organizational structures that were developed in these systems were characterized by decentralization. In larger hospitals, the management for nursing was subdivided with nurse administrators responsible for several patient care units. They reported to the top nurse administrator. Head nurses, known by various titles, reported to these administrators. The head nurse position was considered a key position in these types of structures. Many participating hospitals indicated that educational programs for head nurses had been used to prepare them for their key roles.

Interdepartmental Planning

In addition to restructuring the nursing department, many hospitals reported comprehensive interdepartmental planning to develop efficient systems for maintaining the patient care unit. Planning was coordinated with areas such as housekeeping, materials management and other departments that contributed to maintaining the environment for patient care. Comprehensive planning was also used to develop systems for direct patient services provided by various disciplines. The patient's nurse coordinated the care. Results of this comprehensive planning were improved quality of care and efficiency of all personnel involved, nurses and others. Figure 3 illustrates the relationships between governance, administration, organizational variables, the management unit for nursing and the nursing community that influence nursing care.

Figure 3

Major factors/relationships in organizations that influence nursing practice development.

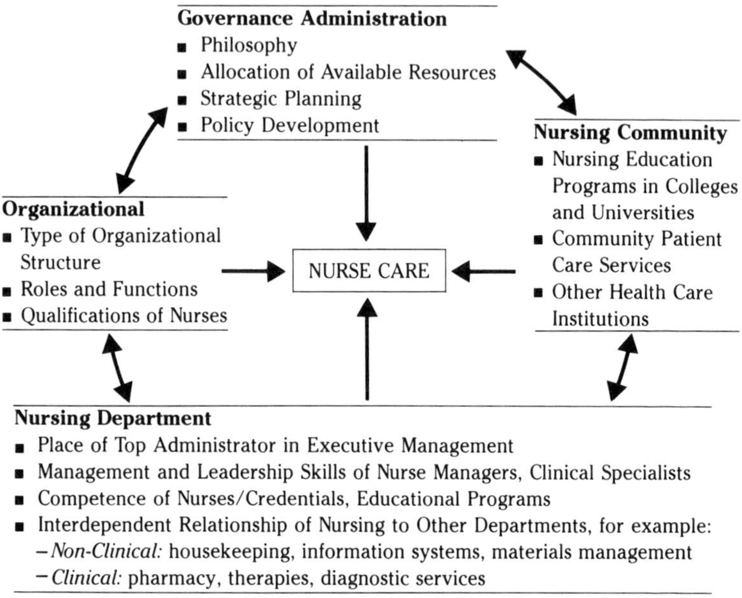

Nursing in Small or Rural Hospitals

A vacancy of only one nurse in a small or rural hospital can be an acute shortage. Characteristics of nursing departments that typify the small or rural hospital were identified in the open forums held in the spring of 1981 in cooperation with the American Hospital Association's Center for Small or Rural Hospitals.

The rural hospital nurse must be a generalist who is able to care for patients with different types of illnesses and all age groups at any given time. Opportunities for the rural hospital nurse are unusual. Considerable autonomy in nursing practice is fostered by the need to incorporate diet therapy, social work, clinical pharmacology, respiratory therapy and other components of care into the nursing role. Ancillary personnel, if available, often serve in a consulting role for short periods of time. The rural hospital nurse has to have a broad knowledge and experience base to provide quality nursing care and has to be a risk taker able to function with minimal supervision.

The versatility inherent in the rural hospital nurses' role is a feature that fosters responsibility and flexibility in nursing practice.

In addition to the unique opportunities for applying the full scope of nursing knowledge in practice, rural hospital nurses enjoy a special place in community life. Close relationships among nurses, physicians, hospital administrators and others allow participative decision making. When these relationships are good, the respect nurses feel in hospital practice is carried over to relationships in the community. If the hospital environment does not support or respect nurses, this lack of respect is reflected back to the community through them and affects nurses' relationships in the community. Nurses in a small community are highly visible and their perceptions of the hospital are a strong influence in the community.

Special problems in recruitment of nurses by small or rural hospitals stem from location and accessibility to schools of nursing and larger health care agencies and the patient population. Small or rural hospitals have limited budgets for recruitment or educational programs such as orientation and staff development. Therefore, major sources of recruitment are the hospital's reputation in the community and the area schools of nursing. Many small or rural hospitals have some form of relationship with a school of nursing: summer work programs for student nurses or arrangements for continuing education that promote improved socialization for nursing students to the rural hospital's unique challenges.

Proximity to larger health care agencies can be both a positive and a negative influence. Accessibility to larger hospitals enables opportunities for nurses to learn about new technology and new equipment used in nursing care. These larger hospitals can, however, draw nurses from a given community if they are willing to commute to the larger center for employment. Consequently, the small hospital suffers the loss.

The patient population in small or rural hospitals appears to be unique in several ways. In general, the patient census tends to fluctuate widely with no apparent pattern. In addition, the patient population appears to be different from patient populations in medical centers. These variations need to be studied to discern the type of educational preparation that would most effectively prepare nurses for rural nursing, ways to utilize these nurses in the community in times of low hospital census and the appropriate mix of nurses and assisting personnel to care for patients.

Some small or rural hospitals have effectively used community resources to encourage recruitment and retention of nurses by finding a job for the nurse's spouse, establishing day care centers or child care options in the community and helping nurses by providing information about state licensure. These hospitals also have worked with area colleges and universities in holding health careers programs or career days and in participating in efforts to bring about legislative changes to benefit potential nursing students. The community visibility of a rural hospital augments these efforts.

In the small community, it is obvious that nurses live in neither a social nor a professional vacuum. If women are opting for careers, then nursing must have proper financial remuneration and recognition to compete with other career opportunities.

A number of issues and problems relating to nursing were seriously addressed in the open forum. As stated by one presenter, "We cannot solve the problem unless we really want to solve the problem. . . unless we work together in a cohesive and intensive effort. . . and commit time, money and other resources to provide the solutions and carry through with them."

Education for Nurse Executives: Report of the Conference, 1981

The commission held an invitational conference attended by representatives of national and regional nursing organizations interested in promoting the development and accessibility of nurse executive educational programs. The participants shared information about the need for such programs and their organization's current programs and resources. A brief summary of description about the participating organizations follows.

Regional Nursing Organizations

NEW ENGLAND COUNCIL OF HIGHER EDUCATION IN NURSING (NECHEN)

The New England Council of Higher Education represents about 58 member educational institutions in six New England states and is a voluntary organization presently supported by the New England Board for Higher Education. A new regional organization to improve collaboration between nursing education and service is being formed. This new organization will be named New England Organization for Nursing (NEON).

MID-ATLANTIC REGIONAL NURSING ASSOCIATION (MARNA)

MARNA is a regional nursing organization formed in July 1981 with membership from the states of Delaware, New Jersey, New York, Pennsylvania and the District of Columbia. Initially funded by a three-year grant from the Division of Nursing, Health and Human Services, MARNA will be supported by agency membership. One of the goals of MARNA is to "foster improvement of administrative skills among nurses in leadership positions."

MIDWEST ALLIANCE IN NURSING (MAIN)

Representing 13 states, MAIN was officially organized in 1979. Partially funded by a W.K. Kellogg Foundation grant, MAIN will be self-supporting by agency membership, with equal representation from nursing education and service on its board and committees. A task group has been appointed to plan for promoting the development of nursing leadership. Needs of the region are being identified to develop a plan.

WESTERN COUNCIL OF HIGHER EDUCATION FOR NURSING (WCHEN)

One of seven programs within the Western Interstate Council of Higher Education (WICHE) representing 13 western states, WCHEN is a consortium of 177 schools of nursing. This quasi-governmental group is funded by both state funds and agency membership. Recently restructured, WCHEN now has two divisions—nursing education and affiliated clinical agencies—and three standing committees. The goals of WCHEN are those of the parent organization: to improve higher education in the West and provide accessibility to education. Unique to WICHE are programs for shared resources through student and faculty exchange.

Advancing collaborative efforts among nurses in education and nursing service settings is one of WCHEN's four main goals. There is particular interest in fostering management team development to meet needs for improved nurse administration, particularly in the rural areas of the West.

THE SOUTHERN COUNCIL ON COLLEGIATE EDUCATION FOR NURSING (SCCEN), SOUTHERN REGIONAL EDUCATIONAL BOARD (SREB)

Representing 14 states, membership of SCCEN consists of regionally accredited colleges and universities with nursing programs. There is an annual membership fee for participating institutions. Serving as a neutral body, SCCEN has been involved in several activities to examine ways to make nurse administrative education accessible. A meeting of representatives of 41 master's programs in nursing from 14 states was held in October 1981; a regional effort for nurse administrator education was favored. Fifteen representatives of nursing service and graduate nursing programs met and decided to hold a regional conference of deans and directors of educational programs and nursing service directors to discuss ways to strengthen and improve accessibility of continuing education and graduate programs in nursing administration.

National Organizations

AMERICAN NURSES' ASSOCIATION (ANA)

The American Nurses' Association's Commission on Nursing Services (now a cabinet) is a council for nursing administration, with more than 300 members and a certification program for nursing administration. The purposes of the council are to:

- promote quality patient care through sound nursing service administration,
- implement ANA standards for nursing services, and
- promote the exchange of ideas.

ANA members with primary interest in and responsibility for enabling and advancing nursing practice organized nursing services are eligible for membership.

Lyndall D. Eddy, R.N., Director, Policy Development and Strategic Planning, is also a co-director of a three-year W.K. Kellogg Foundation funded project to improve management skills of nursing service directors in long-term care facilities. Robert Burmeister, Ph.D., director of the American College of Nursing Home Administrators, Inc. (ACNHA), is co-director.

NATIONAL LEAGUE FOR NURSING (NLN)

The National Forum for Administration of Nursing Services (N-FANS) is a forum for the nurse executive and her/his associates or assistants from acute care, long-term care and community health agencies and graduate level nurse administration courses in educational institutions.

AMERICAN SOCIETY FOR NURSING SERVICE ADMINISTRATORS (ASNSA)

ASNSA advances the development of effective nursing service administration in health care institutions. Educational programs, a Recognition Program for Excellence and other activities support this purpose. The ASNSA has a three-level recognition program for nurse administrators: nominee, candidate and fellow.

DIVISION OF NURSING, AMERICAN HOSPITAL ASSOCIATION

The Division of Nursing provides educational programming and publications related to the practice of nursing service administration, nurse recruitment and retention. In addition, a major division effort centers around informational services to health care managers about issues and problems in nursing that directly affect nursing practice within the individual health care institutions. The division also represents AHA membership concerns in national legislative and regulatory matters.

Resources for Nurse Executive Education

Current resources for nurse executive education were presented at the conference. Presentations were made by representatives of the American Association of Colleges of Nursing, the W.K. Kellogg Foundation, the Minnesota Independent Study Foundation and the Nursing Executive Development Program. A summary of the highlights of these presentations follows.

THE AMERICAN ASSOCIATION OF COLLEGES OF NURSING (AACN)

AACN has examined graduate nursing education in relation to meeting the nation's need for nurses qualified for leadership positions in nursing education, clinical practice, administration and research. In 1981, approximately 50 of the 200 National League for Nursing-accredited higher degree programs offered courses in nursing service administration. Many new programs at the master's and doctoral degree levels are being developed. Trends indicate that emphasis should be placed in developing quality in existing programs. Future development of these programs should take place in educational institutions with a full constellation of health professions, such as in academic health science centers that have the resources needed for quality administration programs. Outreach programs from these major universities are being developed.

Enrollments in nurse administration graduate programs, like other higher educational programs for nursing, are increasing. Part-time students appear to account for a large portion of enrollees. Both the size of the school and faculty qualifications affect quality of programs. Increasing numbers of qualified faculty are needed.

THE DIVISION OF NURSING: HEALTH AND HUMAN SERVICES

The Division of Nursing, Health and Human Services, has stimulated the development of doctoral level programs for nursing service administration.

This development has, through contracts with school, started the process developing model curricula. These schools are the University of Alabama at Birmingham, Indiana University and Boston University.

THE W.K. KELLOGG FOUNDATION

Interdisciplinary graduate nurse administration programs have been supported by the W.K. Kellogg Foundation since 1972. These programs, offered by graduate schools of nursing, cooperate with health service administration programs, business schools and others.

Programs supported by the W.K. Kellogg Foundation are:

Columbia University
School of Public Health
Division of Health Administration
Dr. Lucie Young Kelly

University of Alabama, Birmingham
School of Nursing
Dr. Jean Kelley

University of California, Los Angeles
School of Nursing
Cynthia C. Scalzi

University of Colorado Medical Center
Nursing Service Administrator Program
School of Nursing
Dr. Janelle Krueger

University of Michigan
School of Nursing
Dr. Lillian Simms

University of Minnesota
Program in Public Health Nursing
School of Public Health
Dr. Marla White

University of Pennsylvania
School of Nursing
Dr. Claire M. Fagin

University of Washington
Health Sciences Building
Mrs. Ruth Barney Fine

Virginia Commonwealth University
Medical College of Virginia
Dr. Eleanor Repp

The W.K. Kellogg Foundation also has supported a home study program for practicing directors of nursing services offered by the University of Minnesota Division of Health Services Administration. Support began in 1977. This Independent Study Program in Patient Care Administration provides nursing service administrators with the opportunity to enhance and update their knowledge and skills while remaining in full-time positions.

THE NURSING EXECUTIVE DEVELOPMENT PROGRAM:
AMERICAN HOSPITAL ASSOCIATION:
COLLEGE OF NURSING, UNIVERSITY OF ILLINOIS

This cooperative program was developed to make educational opportunities more accessible to nurse administrators in practice. The American Hospital Association and University of Illinois College of Nursing cooperatively offer the Nurse Executive Development Program. Designed to increase knowledge and skills of nurse executives employed in health care institutions, the program provided flexibility for study within the participant's own organization. Content focuses on patient care and resources and fiscal management organized in 10 independent study modules. Participants also attend residential sessions on campus.

Issues

The outcome of the conference was agreement that both higher degree and continuing education programs for nurse executives need to continue to be developed. Both national and regional acceleration of this development is appropriate. Resources should be consolidated wherever feasible to provide quality educational programs and to maximize use of the limited numbers of qualified nurse faculty available.

Differences between continuing education programs to enhance and update knowledge and skills and degree programs at the master's and doctoral levels should be made clear to enrollees. Both types of programs are needed to fill the current shortage of nurses qualified for administrative roles. As higher degree programs continue to be developed and as practice continues to change, the curriculum should be periodically evaluated to ensure that graduates are prepared for nurse-executive roles and functions.

Credentialing mechanisms such as certification and recognition programs are already in place. Increasingly, the certification and recognition programs are being used in the field for two reasons: to select candidates for nurse executive and management positions and as a measure of institutional quality. These programs are: American Nurses' Association Certification Program for Nursing Administration and American Society for Nursing Service Administrators Recognition Program for Excellence.

Nursing in Multihospital Systems

Invitational Conference: Nursing in Multihospital Systems

The commission's national conference about nursing in multihospital systems was held in early 1982 to examine the roles and functions of nurses employed at the corporate level in multihospital systems and the influence of multihospital systems on hospital nursing practice. The discussion at this conference covered topics of corporate nursing roles and functions and features of multihospital systems that had particular implications for nurse administrators. Resource availability, flexibility, standardization, communication and systemwide policies were discussed.

Education, employment, standards for quality research, technology, finance and corporate-community relationships were areas of corporate level involvement with nursing identified by nurses at the conference. Twelve corporations were represented by 15 nurses who either held corporate level positions for nursing or represented corporations. Investor-owned and not-for-profit corporations were represented.

Discussion began with two questions: How is the nursing function conceived and organized at the corporate level? and What is the projected long-term influence of multihospital systems on nursing? By the end of the conference, it was clear that corporations had an interest in nursing issues and problems and that there was variation in the ways nursing in member hospitals related to the corporation. It was agreed that a survey was needed to further explore these relationships and the new type of nursing leader that will be needed by corporations in the future.

This survey was conducted in November/December 1982. Results of the survey are in Appendix 1.

Bibliography

American Association of Colleges of Nursing. Descriptive brochure of the AACN. Washington, D.C.: The Association, 1981.

American Nurses' Association—Commission on Nursing Education. *Funding Nursing Education.* Publication No. NE-7 5-M, Kansas City, MO: The Association, 1980.

American Nurses' Association—Commission on Nursing Education. *Statement on Graduate Education in Nursing.* Kansas City, MO: The Association, 1981.

American Nurses' Association—Commission on Nursing Services. *Roles, Responsibilities, and Qualifications for Nurse Administrators.* Publication No. NS-23 3M. Kansas City, MO: The Association, 1978.

American Nurses' Association—Statement of Task Force on a Nursing Professional Climate. *Characteristics of a Professional Climate of Administration and Practice in a Nursing Department.* Kansas City, MO: The Association, 1979.

Murphy, Marion I. *Master's Programs in Nursing in the Eighties: Trends and Issues.* Washington, D.C.: American Association of Colleges of Nursing, 1981.

National League for Nursing—Council of Baccalaureate and Higher Degree Programs. *Master's Education in Nursing: Route to Opportunities in Contemporary Nursing,* 1981-82. New York: The League, 1981.

National League for Nursing—Council of Baccalaureate and Higher Degree Programs. *Doctoral Programs in Nursing,* 1981-82. New York: The League, 1982.

Slater, C.H. *The Education and Roles of Nursing Service Administrators.* Battle Creek, MI: W.K. Kellogg Foundation, 1978.

Smith, M.H. *Graduate Education in Nursing: Issues and Future Directions.* Atlanta: Southern Regional Educational Board, 1981.

University of Minnesota—School of Public Health. Independent Study Program in Patient Care Administration, Department of Independent Study of Continuing Education and Extension at the University of Minnesota (developed in 1973).

Chapter 5

THE NURSING PROFESSION

Information pertaining to the nursing profession is presented in this section in two different areas: nursing's professional organizations and credentialing in nursing. Both of these topics reflect nursing's involvement in efforts to ensure the qualifications of nurses in practice.

Nursing is in transition. Nursing functions in the 1980s are different from those in the 1960s. The environment of health care, the technology of patient care and the knowledge base and complexity of patient care needs are changing. In hospitals, for example, the acuity of illness and consequently the intensity of patient care have increased. Similar influences have been felt by nurses practicing in other settings.

Different perceptions about nursing were expressed in the extensive and thoughtful reviews of the commission's *Initial Report and Preliminary Recommendations*. There is a need for common understanding about nursing.

The various nursing professional organizations have been formed over time to develop the processes needed to sustain nursing's ability to provide high-quality patient care. Some of these organizations have their origins in nursing's early development in the United States. Others have more recently been formed in response to increasing clinical specialization.

Results of the commission's 1982 survey of nursing organizations are given in Appendix 2. Several of these organizations have nurse credentialing programs. Credentialing is part of the total effort to differentiate for the public who a nurse is and what nurses are qualified to do in practice.

Credentialing in Nursing

The need to distinguish among nurses by level of education and performance capabilities was established in testimony at the public hearings and responses to the *Initial Report and Preliminary Recommendations*. This need is expected to become more acute as health care becomes more complex and costs are constrained. It is projected that fewer but more highly qualified nurses will be needed in this system. Both nurses and employers will benefit from a clear credentialing system that allows them to distinguish among various nurses' performance capabilities. This credentialing system will promote efficiency in education, employment and practice to ensure basic qualifications and provide for recognition of nurses' expertise in practice.

In credentialing, as in other aspects of nursing, transition to the future must evolve from the present for long-lasting improvement. Adding new dimensions without developing present resources may be temporarily useful but difficult to sustain over time. Currently, nursing has various credentialing processes in place. Some of these are newly forming, such as certification programs for individual nurses, while others have a longer history of development, such as licensure and accreditation. Efforts have been ongoing in nursing to relate these programs in a more comprehensive system that will be easily understood and helpful to nurses and the patients they serve.

Definition of Credentialing

"Credentialing refers to the processes by which individuals or institutions, or one or more of their programs, are designated by a qualified agent as having met minimum standards at a specified time."[1] This definition includes the inextricably related credentialing processes of academic degrees and diplomas, licensing, registration, certification, accreditation, approval and recognition. Credentialing may be voluntary or mandatory, private or governmental and may denote quality, confer identity, provide protection and/or serve as an instrument of control. Credentialing processes in nursing fulfill the mandate to protect the public health, safety and welfare, as well as to protect the title and practice of nurses.[2] Definitions of credentialing processes used by the American Nurses' Association credentialing study committee are shown in Tables 1 and 2.

Various credentialing processes in nursing are in different stages of development. Licensure, which is conferred by states under statutory authority, was the earliest development. The first Nurse Practice Act in the United States was passed in North Carolina in 1903, and by 1923, all states had licensure laws. Licensure is mandatory for nursing practice in 48 states and the District of Columbia. Nursing has enjoyed a relatively uniform system for nurse licensure throughout the United States. Model Nurse Practice Acts are available from two sources: the American Nurses' Association and the National Council on State Boards of Nursing, Inc. Each state and the District of Columbia may use these acts as guides in implementation of their own stat-

---

[1] American Nurses' Association. *The Study of Credentialing in Nursing: A New Approach*. Vol. 1, Code G-1365M, Report of the Committee. Kansas City, MO, March 1979.

[2] Styles, M. Credentialing issues in nursing. Unpublished paper presented to National Commission on Nursing, 1982.

Table 1

Definitions of credentialing processes for individuals and institutional programs.

Educational Degrees	An academic degree is a title awarded to an individual who has successfully taken an officially recognized, predetermined series of steps in a particular branch of learning. The designation of the degree signifies the level of education and indicates an arts or science area. The professional degree is similar but the designation differs in indicating the specific professional field of study.
Licensure	A process by which an agency of state government grants permission to individuals accountable for the practice of a profession to engage in the practice of that profession and prohibits all others from legally doing so. It permits use of a particular title. Its purpose is to protect the public by ensuring a minimum level of professional competence. Established standards and methods of evaluation are used to determine eligibility for initial licensure and for periodic renewal. Effective means are employed for taking action against licensees for acts of professional misconduct, incompetence and/or negligence.
Registration	A process by which qualified individuals are listed on an official roster maintained by a governmental or non-governmental agency. It enables such persons to use a particular title and attests to employing agencies and individuals that minimum qualifications have been met and maintained.
Certification	A process by which a non-governmental agency or association certifies that an individual licensed to practice a profession has met certain predetermined standards specified by that profession for specialty practice. Its purpose is to assure various publics that an individual has mastered a body of knowledge and acquired skills in a particular specialty.
Recognition	A process whereby one agency or association accepts for specified purposes the credentialing status of and the credentials conferred by another credentialing body.

utes as appropriate. Licensure legalizes basic nursing practice as indicated to ensure an acceptable level of quality.

Elements commonly found in State Nurse Practice Acts are:

- a definition of nursing practice;
- criteria for licensure;
- conditions under which licenses can be revoked or suspended;
- approval of nursing education programs;
- provisions for formulation of roles and regulations to implement the Nurse Practice Act; and
- designation of authority to persons to administer the statute through administrative processes of state government, most often by a state board of nursing or its equivalent.

Table 2

Definitions of credentialing processes for institutions.

Approval	A process whereby one agency assesses the practices of another agency for consistency of procedural practices and for evidence of integrity in its conduct of business.
Accreditation	The process by which a voluntary, non-governmental agency or organization appraises and grants accredited status to institutions and/or programs or services which meet predetermined structure, process and outcome criteria. Its purposes are to evaluate the performance of a service or educational program and to provide to various publics information upon which to base decisions about the utilization of the institutions, programs, services and/or graduates. Periodic assessment is an integral part of the accreditation process in order to ensure continual acceptable performance. Accreditation is conducted by agencies which have been recognized or approved by an organized peer group of agencies as having integrity and consistency in their practices.
Charter	The mechanism by which an agency of state government, under the laws of the state, grants corporate existence to an institution with or without the right to award degrees.

The Licensure Examination

The National Council of State Boards, Inc. contracts for the preparation of the nurse licensure examination that is administered in all states twice a year. The National Council Licensure examination (formerly called the State Board Test Pool Exam) is owned and directed by the National Council of State Boards, Inc. In 1982, the Council administered a new, integrated examination with one overall score. Previously, the state board examination had consisted of five separately scored examinations in areas of medical nursing, surgical nursing, psychiatric nursing, nursing of children and obstetric nursing. In July 1982, criterion-referenced scoring of the examination was initiated, replacing the traditional norm-referenced scoring. Successfully passing the licensure examination is one criterion for licensure.[3]

Approval of Nursing Education Programs

In most states, individual licensure is contingent on successful completion of a state-approved nursing education program. All 50 states and the District of Columbia have nursing programs in junior and senior colleges and universities. Thirty-eight states also have hospital schools of nursing. Approval (called accreditation in some states) of nursing programs is authorized by the Nurse Practice Act and, as such, is under governmental purview and often is limited to prelicensure educational programs.

[3] Dvorak, E. National Council of State Boards of Nursing. Presentation to National Commission on Nursing, 1982.

Precedent for using curriculum standards as a requirement for licensure eligibility can be traced to the early New York Nurse Practice Act. It required that nurses seeking licensure in New York be graduated from schools of nursing with curriculums approved by the Regents of the University of the State of New York. This provision had the effect of standardizing curricula throughout the United States so that nursing school graduates could obtain reciprocity in New York state.

A current issue in approval of nursing education programs is that governmental approval of schools of nursing may infringe on academic freedom and duplicate voluntary accreditation processes. The fundamental purpose of approval is to ensure that graduates have completed a nursing curriculum that prepares them adequately for nursing practice.

Accreditation of Nursing Education Programs

Voluntary accreditation of nursing programs began in 1939 through the National League for Nursing Education and earlier by the National Organization for Public Health Nursing and the Council on Nursing Education of the Catholic Hospital Association of the United States and Canada. In 1948, accreditation was centralized in the National Nursing Accrediting Service. Accreditation was designated as a function of the newly formed National League for Nursing in 1952.[4]

Voluntary accreditation by the NLN is now available for basic nursing education programs and master's degree programs in nursing. The National League for Nursing has "deemed status" from the Health Standards and Quality Bureau, Health Care Financing Administration. Recently, the NLN completed a major study of accreditation policies and procedures, and implementation of its recommendations is under way.

Accreditation of Continuing Education

The American Nurses' Association provides accreditation for continuing education programs in nursing. It began this accreditation program in 1974. Some state nurses' associations also have continuing education program approval processes, as do some state boards of nursing. A number of states have mandatory continuing education for relicensure as indicated in Table 3.

Certification and Recognition for Nurses

Both certification and recognition processes are voluntary and are designed to ensure qualifications for specialty nursing practice in various clinical specialties, such as critical care nursing or in functional areas such as administration. Certification and recognition programs are relatively new in their present form. The American Nurses' Association has 17 different certification programs and many specialty organizations have certification programs for

---

[4] Styles, M. Credentialing issues in nursing. Unpublished paper presented to National Commission on Nursing, 1982.

Table 3

States having mandatory continuing education (CE) for nurses, 1981.

[Twelve (23.5 percent) states have mandatory CE for RNs]
[Four (7.8 percent) states have mandatory CE for nurse practitioners only]

Alaska	Mandatory for Nurse Practitioners only
California	Mandatory
Colorado	Mandatory
Florida	Mandatory
Indiana	Requires Standards of Practice; not CE
Iowa	Mandatory
Kansas	Mandatory
Kentucky	Mandatory
Massachusetts	Mandatory
Minnesota	Mandatory
Mississippi	Mandatory for Nurse Practitioners only
Nebraska	Mandatory
Nevada	Mandatory
New Hampshire	Mandatory for Nurse Practitioners only
New Mexico	Mandatory
North Carolina	Proposal Stage as of March 1981
Washington	Mandatory
Puerto Rico	Mandatory

their given specialty area. Most of these programs use similar criteria: educational preparation, current experience in the area of practice, validation of excellence or standards of performance and successful completion of an examination. As certification is increasingly used in the selection of candidates for certain positions in nursing practice and as the complexity of patient care increases, the master's degree is becoming a recommended, if not required, criterion in some certification programs. This trend is reflected in some state laws pertaining to advanced specialty nursing practice.

Various certification programs in nursing have been developed independently by different nursing organizations, resulting in some overlapping, some competition and a scope ranging from ensuring basic performance to recognizing excellence in a given specialty. Nurses, however, are increasingly seeking means for recognition of excellence in practice and are looking to professional certification as a means to validate their achievement. Current recognition and certification programs are a mechanism to enable nurses with varied educational preparation to demonstrate their competence. Employers of nurses are beginning to use certification as a means for selecting the most qualified nurses for leadership positions, particularly in clinical specialties and administration.

Governmental

States, through a variety of means such as licensure or certification, and agencies, such as departments of health or consumer affairs or others, approve health care institutions and programs, including the nursing services within them.[5]

Voluntary

The National League for Nursing offers an accreditation program for community nursing services and home health agencies. Nursing services in hospitals are included within the scope of Joint Commission on Accreditation of Hospitals accreditation. The American Nurses' Association is working toward cooperative efforts to set the standards for evaluation of nursing within this process, as well as to gain a designated seat or seats upon the board of this jointly established hospital accrediting body.

Study of Credentialing

The American Nurses' Association completed a study of credentialing in nursing in 1979.[6] One of the recommendations of the study was to establish a freestanding national nursing credentialing center to achieve a unified, coordinated, comprehensive credentialing system for nursing. A resolution to implement this recommendation was passed by the ANA in 1982.

Summary of Issues and Future Actions

A broad issue in credentialing is how to provide an efficient system of credentialing that allows state governments and the nursing profession to meet their respective accountabilities to the public.

Purposes of credentialing are to protect public health, safety and welfare and to protect the title and/or practice of the individual. Certification and recognition programs that provide for rigorous evaluation of performance capability can benefit both the public and the individual seeking recognition in a nursing career. State governments have the legal authority to license nurses for practice for the purpose of protecting the public by ensuring an acceptable level of competence. The nursing profession determines the standards for basic and advanced nursing practice.

Many groups, including nurses, public policymakers, employers of nurses and patients, are looking to nursing to provide them with valid indicators of a given nurse's capability for quality performance in patient care.

---

[5] Styles, M. Credentialing issues in nursing. Unpublished paper presented to National Commission on Nursing, 1982.

[6] American Nurses' Association. *The Study of Credentialing in Nursing: A New Approach.* Vol. 1, Code G-1365M, Report of the Committee. Kansas City, MO, March 1979.

They are seeking the means to distinguish the most qualified nurses to provide the increasingly complex technologic nursing care required in today's health care system.

Nurses in practice, education, administration, research and public policy have a role to play in keeping nursing knowledge and practice up to date. They can cooperatively develop new knowledge and practice skills that will be needed. In this effort, nursing can effectively retain the strong element of caring that characterizes nursing, as well as sustain the standards and mechanisms for monitoring nursing competence. The increased rate of growth of patient care knowledge and technology requires that nurses cooperate in establishing educational and practice structures with credentialing processes that are appropriate to the future.

In making the transition to the future, nursing needs to assess its current credentialing system for its capability to recognize competent nurses already in practice. Vision is needed for continued development of existing credentialing processes to ensure that continued upgrading of curricula and corresponding upgrading of credentialing criteria and examination content reflect more complex roles and functions of nurses. Attention to the effectiveness, efficiency and visibility of nursing's credentialing system is needed now and will continue to be needed in the future to ensure quality nursing care.

Chapter

6

NURSING EDUCATION

"The site of an educational program is not absolute. What is fundamental is that any site be conducive to and supportive in space, appointments equipment, supplies and environment of quality education; that the curriculum offered be of academic excellence and that the faculty imparting the knowledge bear the university/college appointment imprimatur in all dimensions of the degree-awarding institution as to teaching competence. Faculty appointments should be awarded only after rigorous review and evaluation of credentials and certification of performance."

Matthew McNulty
Chancellor
The Medical Center
Georgetown University

In the long run, decisions about nursing education will be influenced by patients seeking quality nursing care. As an independent body, the commission was able to step back from the acute manifestations of change to obtain an overall view of nursing education. The long-range view identified was one of gradual but persistent change, occurring at an uneven rate across the United States, but with a clearly defined direction to upgrading nursing education (Figure 4). Nursing education is in transition. The pace and geographic variations in the transition can be related as much to the historical status of primary, secondary and higher education in different regions as to the status of women and other societal factors. The movement to advance nursing education can be related primarily to increased complexity of patient care.

The commission's education committee deliberated the issues of transition. A summary of the committee's explication of the route to the future is presented in this section.

Figure 4

Educational sequence for upward mobility for registered nurses.

Doctoral Degree (PhD, Doctorate in Nursing Science)* for Advanced Clinical, Administrative, Teaching and Research Roles

Master's in Nursing Degree for Clinical Specialization, Administration, Teaching and Research Roles

Baccalaureate in Nursing Degree for General Professional Practice

Associate Degree/Diploma

* There is also entry to professional nursing at the generic master's and nursing doctorate program.

Future goals for nursing require:

- education in institutions of higher learning;
- graduate level education for teaching, research and administrative and public service roles; and
- established standards for education, licensure and certification.

These future goals are long-range. Currently, nursing is in transition to reach these future goals. It is important during this transition to maintain the quality of patient care and to ensure that the individuals currently in nursing have opportunities to maintain and upgrade their own status according to their capabilities and desires.

There currently exists a large number of nurses prepared in various types of nursing educational programs and located in different kinds of institutions. During the transition, recognition must be given to: need for an increased number of nurses; maintenance of an adequate number of nurses; adherence to an acceptable level of patient care during the transition; and maintenance of reasonable cost of nursing care to the public.

There are four main areas for consideration in planning for accelerating the transition of nursing education into the mainstream of higher education:

- planning on a regional/statewide basis;
- educational resources;
- protection of individuals; and
- relationships between nursing education and practice.

Planning on a Regional and Statewide Basis

Regional or statewide planning is an appropriate way to balance resources and needs for nursing education. In each region or state, existing educational resources that need to be adapted to the nursing education system of the future differ. Additional short-term funding may be needed to support transition efforts. Some aspects of state planning to be considered are:

- nursing's professional associations should play the major role in planning with health professionals from other disciplines and appropriate government agencies participating;

- plans should be targeted to specific objectives, and there should be progress reports and evaluation of outcomes achieved;
- dissemination of information about effective state planning already accomplished or under way should promote sharing and cooperation among institutions and states;
- transitional educational programs in state plans should provide opportunity for nurses in practice according to their goals and ability in nursing; and
- statewide planning should be synchronized with developments in nursing knowledge and the upgraded technology needed for nursing care.

Educational Resources

Existing educational resources should be used in the transition to collegiate degree-based educational programs by:

- conducting joint efforts of hospitals, colleges and universities through cooperation, collaboration, charter or other institutional options to develop nursing programs in the system of higher education;
- maintaining standards for accreditation of educational programs that are appropriately flexible in their application to programs attempting to convert to baccalaureate education; and
- devising additional standards that may need to be outlined for collaborative efforts.

In addition, successful models of education that maintain standards, promote transition and ensure an adequate supply of nurses should be publicized and information about their operation should be disseminated. Attention also must be given to the preparation of nurse-administrators of both education and practice institutions as key to establishing future education and practice settings. Education at the graduate level should include both clinical and management content necessary for credibility and quality patient care.

Protection of Individuals

Current licensure status of registered nurses with associate degrees or diplomas should be protected as standards are upgraded. When the transition is completed, all nurses entering nursing should meet the new standards. Registered nurses who wish to complete baccalaureate and higher degrees should have a clear sequence of educational opportunities. Financial support of both educational institutions and students from all sources, including the employment setting, should be targeted to support professional nurses in baccalaureate and higher degree education. Graduate education is critical to developing the leadership cadre necessary for the education and practice of professional nursing.

Relationships Between Nursing Education and Practice

To ensure quality patient care, professional nurses should be prepared in clinical nursing educational programs in colleges and universities. Nursing education and practice should be reciprocally related in the development of the knowledge base and in practice. The synergy resulting from good education-practice relationships should vitalize nursing. Attention should be given to the clinical nursing component of educational programs and the way education relates to practice. The linkage between nursing education and practice should promote early inclusion of new knowledge and technology from practice into education and new knowledge from faculty research into practice.

Both basic research and clinical research are key to continued development of nursing knowledge and technology underlying quality patient care.

Differentiation of Nurses

Confusion about nursing education and practice stemming from lack of differentiation among nurses was reported as a problem in the commission's public hearings and in responses to the preliminary recommendations. A title for nurses that would clearly identify categories of nurses by their educational preparation, experience, proved performance and professional contribution was thought essential to clearing up the confusion about nursing.

Credentialing

Opportunities for eligible registered nurses from associate degree and diploma programs to enter baccalaureate degree and higher degree programs should be promoted. The experience and the quality of performance should distinguish the qualifications among nurses.

Current issues in credentialing include: problems in changing the state statutes for nurse licensure; the possibility of establishing voluntary certification by examination or other means for nurses with baccalaureate degrees to determine advanced competence of these nurses; or establishing an additive credential for nurses with baccalaureate and higher degrees to become certified baccalaureate degree nurses. To understand more about nursing departments and schools of nursing, the commission conducted a survey of nursing education in hospitals. A report on this survey is contained in Appendix 5.

Chapter 7

POLICY AND THE ENVIRONMENT FOR NURSING PRACTICE

The National Commission on Nursing's recommendations have implications for policy at institutional, local, state and national levels. Research grounded in understanding the causes and effects of nursing-related events is needed as a base for policy decisions. The commission's recommendations were developed from an analytic framework that can serve as a research perspective for evaluation and development of research. The key relationships identified in this framework are of particular importance to the commission's work. Key relationships between nursing and institutions, other health professionals, nursing organizations and the public, and the relationship between nursing education and nursing practice are all inextricably related. They all contribute to the nursing practice environment and the expectations nurses have for that environment.

Research is needed to improve the existing knowledge base for future policy decisions. This section contains information about research related to the organizational role of the nurse and the nursing practice environment. The supplemental report of the survey of innovative programs and projects contains the results of a survey conducted by the commission about research related to this topic.

The Organizational Role of the Hospital Nurse: Synthesis of Research and A Proposed Model

by Jeffrey A. Alexander, Ph.D.

Introduction

The research literature reviewed in this paper has as its focus the organizational role of the hospital nurse. As an outcome of this review, the paper offers a set of policy recommendations and proposes an analytic framework for examining the relationship between hospital organizational structure/process and organizational outcomes relevant to nursing.

Four assumptions underlie the choice of the hospital organization as the context for examining nursing roles and outcomes:

- Many of the highly publicized problems surrounding nursing today, such as nursing shortages, high turnover and work stoppages, are symptomatic rather than causal in nature. Investigations that have focused only on these symptoms have shed little light on their causal antecedents. The adoption of a single, organizational perspective on nursing issues allows the specification of common linkages between problems and provides a basis for understanding rather than mere description of the issues.
- Much of the current discussion and research on nursing problems has focused on solutions that would alter the supply and education of nurses in the future, with little attention given to the situation of nurses currently working in the health care system. Because over 60 percent of active nurses are employed in hospitals, an organizational perspective that examines the problems nurses experience in practice is highly appropriate to developing a comprehensive understanding of nursing issues.
- Existing literature on nursing suggests that many nursing issues are affected by multiple *processes* and *participants* in the health care system. Because hospitals represent the focus of activity for many of these elements, including physicians, administrators and patients, it is particularly appropriate to examine nursing issues at this interface.
- Identification of nursing issues in the context of the hospital organization offers the potential of formulating interventions that are relevant to the nurse in her/his arena of practice and amenable to implementation by individual hospital and nursing administrators. This organizational perspective complements the national policy emphasis of manpower and education studies on nursing, which does not address effectively the immediate concerns of those who must face nursing-related problems on a day-to-day basis.

Jeffrey A. Alexander, Ph.D., is senior researcher at the Hospital Research and Educational Trust and directs the Trust's Office of Organizational Studies.

Review of Research on Hospital Nursing Literature: An Organizational Perspective

Overview

A major review of the nursing literature conducted by the Department of Health, Education and Welfare Division of Nursing (Jelinek and Dennis 1976) concludes that despite the plethora of studies relating the role of the hospital nurse and the organization of hospital nursing services, few of these studies are well designed, well executed or conclusive in their findings. The absence of a solid theoretical framework is seen as a major contributor to inconsistency in measuring and inaccuracy in defining factors that affect the nurse's role in the hospital. This limitation is, in part, a function of the complex and sometimes conflicting context in which nursing is performed. Differences in perspectives on the nursing function occur among nurses, administrators and physicians, and the complex organizational arrangements under which nurses work make a unified research framework difficult. The resulting character of nursing research has been a narrow focus on subsets of organizational issues with only limited attempts to relate findings to other areas of investigation.

This review attempts to develop an integrated research perspective on the nurse in the hospital organization. Because of the fragmented state of the literature, an inductive approach to this task is adopted. Specifically, research related to organizational outcomes relevant to nursing are considered. This review focuses on sets of empirical determinants that suggest processes and conditions under which such outcomes occur. The second part of the review develops conceptual explanations underlying these potential causal processes and serves as the foundation for a general model of nursing outcomes in hospitals.

Nurses in Hospitals—Organizational Outcomes

Two organizational outcomes relevant to problems in hospital nursing are treated extensively in the literature: turnover and collective bargaining. In addition, several intermediate outcomes relevant to hospital nursing are considered, including job satisfaction, role conflict and alienation. It has been argued previously that such phenomena are probably manifestations of problems rather than problems in themselves. However, a review of the literature in these related areas may yield categories of organizational variables that suggest underlying issues.

Determinants of turnover, collective bargaining and intermediate nursing outcomes can be classified under three general headings: job content, job context and individual attributes. Job content refers to structural characteristics of tasks performed by the individual nurse: role, organizational position, specialization or formalization. Job context includes organizational characteristics at the level of the hospital or immediate work group, such as coordination and control, decision-making practices, evaluation mechanisms or supervisory style.

These two categories are similar because they emphasize the organizational rather than technological nature of nursing work. They differ primarily in the level of analysis of those organizational features—individual or group, a distinction that is often blurred in the literature.

The third category of determinants, individual attributes, refers to personal characteristics of the nurse, such as age, marital status, job tenure and number of children.

This taxonomy differs from that found in earlier research on nursing which often grouped determinants of nursing behavior/attitudes into categories of intrinsic and extrinsic rewards. Such a classification scheme is exclusively behavioral in character and does not recognize organizational or social determinants of nursing behavior.

Turnover

Turnover may be defined as the number of workers in an organization who voluntarily leave their jobs during a specified period of time. High turnover and inactivity rates among nurses are of direct relevance to the nursing shortage issue and of immediate concern to hospital administrators faced with problems of staffing and cost containment. Hospital costs associated with recruitment and hiring, personnel orientation and training have been shown to increase as a function of high turnover (Sloan 1975, Kase and Swenson 1976). Turnover also has been associated with diminished productivity and nursing effectiveness (Burlington et al 1956, Revans 1964).

Much of the literature in this area has attempted to examine the relationship between job satisfaction and rates of turnover. This literature has been limited in its ability to explain turnover and its attendant, job satisfaction, for several reasons. First, it has relied primarily on the self reports of nurses who have resigned, thereby introducing biases inherent to retrospective research designs—recall and cognitive dissonance. Further, these designs have typically not included a comparison group of nurses who remain in the hospital. Thus, it cannot be ascertained whether the determinants of turnover are more or less equally distributed between these two groups. Another weakness of such research is its emphasis on bivariate analysis techniques; that is, looking only at one set of potential causal variables. This design results in an inadequate accounting of alternative explanations of the turnover phenomenon (Campbell and Stanley 1963).

Traditionally, turnover and job satisfaction among nurses have been attributed to individual attributes such as marital status, short job tenure and first job incumbency (Sloan 1975, Seybolt et al 1978, Knopf 1975, Kramer 1974). In a related vein, personal correlates of job satisfaction among nurses and women in general have included type of education, number of children and degree of perceived internal control. Other studies, however, suggest that reasons for turnover pertain to job-related factors rather than to personal factors (Diamond and Fox 1958, Saleh et al 1965, USVA 1973, McCloskey 1974).

Self-reported organizational or job-related reasons for turnover include overtime work, rotating shifts, high work load, poor nurse leadership, poor relations with physicians and inadequate time for professional development (McCloskey 1974, Seybolt et al 1978, McClure 1972, Brief 1976, Everly and Falcione 1976). Relatively few studies, however, have examined such organizational attributes in an objective fashion. One of the few exceptions is the work of Munson and Heda (1974), which related direct measures of unit work load and staffing patterns with level of satisfaction among hospital nurses. More recently, a study by Weisman et al (1980) employed multivariate analysis and direct indicators to examine a theoretical model relating nurse turnover to job satisfaction, propensity to leave, autonomy and sets of organizational and individual characteristics. A multivariate analysis attempts to account for a number of affecting factors simultaneously. They found that the strongest predictors of nurses' job satisfaction were organizational in nature, followed by structural attributes of units and individual characteristics of nurses. Weisman's study is particularly notable as it is one of the few that employs multivariate analysis and a prospective design.

Kramer and Baker (1971), in a prospective study of 223 baccalaureate nurses, noted that nurses who did not relinquish their professional values during hospital employment were prone to leave nursing even though they may have been labeled as successful by their employer. Role conflict engendered by the incompatability of nurses' professional values and hospital bureaucracy was cited as the explanation for exiting.

McCloskey (1974) supported these findings in his examination of 94 nurses. His findings indicated that although nurses are drawn to a job because of extrinsic rewards, such as salary and working conditions, they tend to leave because of lack of intrinsic rewards, such as professional self-actualization.

Lyons (1970), Dauw (1966), and Behling and Kosmo (1971) investigated the turnover phenomenon using a multivariate framework. Lyons (1970), for example, posited that role clarity, organizational communication and coordination, and job tension should be related to each other and to turnover. His results suggest that turnover is inversely related to satisfaction and role clarity, and directly related to tension and inadequate communication and coordination.

In a later investigation of 105 nursing units in two metropolitan hospitals, Weisman et al (1980) examined the effects of individual characteristics, structural attributes of nursing units and job characteristics on turnover. A causal model was developed that linked perceived autonomy to job satisfaction which, in turn, affected intent to leave and ultimately turnover among registered nurses. High autonomy was associated with longer length of employment, working a permanent shift, higher position level and less overtime. Job satisfaction was determined to be a critical variable in predicting intent to leave. Salary and demographic characteristics, such as marriage and child rearing were not found to be significant in this causal model. Based on their findings Weisman et al (1980) recommend increasing task integrity and administrative autonomy of nurses, increasing unit staffing levels and decreasing work load as administrative interventions that may reduce nursing turnover.

Finally, in another prospective investigation, Price and Mueller (1981) examined turnover rates among 1,091 register nurses employed in seven hospitals. Findings of the study indicated that low routinization, high instrumental communication, high promotional opportunity and high participation in decision making all contribute to job satisfaction which, in turn, affects turnover. The study further pointed out that extrinsic rewards such as salary are not significant determinants in the causal model. Price and Mueller suggest that the professional orientation of registered nurses may cause a deemphasis on the value of pay for these individuals and that nurses emphasize job content and job context characteristics to a greater extent.

The findings from the literature on nurse turnover suggest that extrinsic rewards play little part in a nurse's decision to leave the profession. More important are the organizational constraints associated with the job and certain individual attributes, such as job and occupational tenure. This body of research is useful insofar as it identifies broad categories of determinants of nursing turnover. However, the methodological and conceptual weaknesses of most work on nursing turnover renders its usefulness for policy development questionable.

An intermediate outcome that has been closely linked to nursing turnover is job satisfacton. Price (1972:156) defines job satisfaction as the degree to which members of a social system have a positive orientation toward membership in that system. Research on both turnover and job satisfaction attempts to isolate the determinants that best predict these outcomes. Research on job satisfaction, however, typically employs theoretical orientations specific to psychology (e.g., Maslow, Herzberg), while the turnover literature assumes predominantly a socio-psychological perspective. The job satisfaction literature on nursing lacks strong theoretical and methodological substance. These difficulties are manifested in poorly developed measures of the concept of job satisfaction and in the lack of meaningful taxonomies of the determinants of job satisfaction. Given these weaknesses, it is not surprising that the findings in this area have been largely inconclusive. Studies that suggest that factors related to salary and working conditions (extrinsic factors) are associated with job satisfaction are as prevalent as studies that argue the importance of intrinsic characteristics of nursing (Marlow 1966, Benton and White 1972, White and McGuire 1973, Bullough 1974).

In one of the few strong investigations, Weisman et al (1980) conducted a longitudinal analysis of job satisfaction among hospital nurses. Examined in the study were both organizational and nonorganizational determinants of job satisfaction. Results of the analysis for nurses employed in 105 units in two major metropolitan hospitals indicated that the strongest predictors of nursing satisfaction were organizational in nature, followed by structural attributes and finally by individual characteristics of nurses. Weisman and her colleagues concluded that nurses were satisfied with their jobs if they perceived that they controlled their work through independent decision making and if physicians did not delegate inappropriate tasks to them.

A major contribution of the job satisfaction literature is the conceptualization of job satisfaction among nurses as multidimensional in nature (e.g., working conditions, professional relationships, authority and decision making). Given the complexity of nursing functions and roles in the hospital, such a multidimensional approach to job satisfaction is particularly appropriate (Everly and Falcione 1976).

Collective Bargaining

Collective bargaining between hospital administration and staff nurses occurs relatively infrequently. The literature on collective bargaining is consequently sparse relative to that on turnover and job satisfaction. However, to the extent that collective bargaining can be construed as symptomatic of organizational problems affecting both nurses and hospitals, an examination of this literature is warranted.

Much of the early work on collective bargaining (Kravit 1973, Grand 1973) discusses it in terms of the shift in professional ideology that nursing has experienced over the past 20 years. Collective bargaining is seen by Grand (1973), for example, as an ideology of "professional collectivism" whereby nurses express public criticism of the quality of patient care to legitimize their dissatisfaction with salary and working conditions.

Several studies have focused on defining and testing the determinants of collective action among nurses (Meyer 1968, Bloom et al 1980, Alutto and Balasco 1972). These studies are valuable insofar as they generate evidence about organizational sources of dissatisfaction and may thus provide administrators with guidelines for alleviating problems leading to collective bargaining situations.

Meyer (1968) constructed and tested a behavioral model of collective action attitudes among hospital nurses. His findings indicated significant relationships between frustrated desires for autonomy and the predisposition toward collective action. Bloom et al (1980) examined the collective bargaining attitudes of 78 staff nurses and 11 supervisory nurses engaged in public health activity. Both striking and nonstriking nurses were interviewed and determinants of strike behavior were examined using factor and multivariate analysis. The investigators found that perceptions of the striking nurses differed from those of management on nearly half of the 17 issues under consideration. While management felt that industrial sector bargaining issues, such as wages and job security, were critical problems for the nurses, the nurses were more concerned with matters related to communication with management and participation in organizational decision making.

Over a six year period, Management Science Associates surveyed 110,000 hospital workers, including 20,000 registered nurses, about attitudes and opinions relating to unions and collective bargaining (Stickler and Velghe 1980). Nurses were surveyed before and after union representation elections and in hospitals where there was no union activity. Analysis of the survey suggests that the role of the professional nurse in the hospital is not meeting nurses' job needs. Factors associated with disposition to unionize included: need for more individual freedom in the performance of nursing tasks; need for greater input in job-related matters; need for greater control over work schedule; and a more flexible management approach in dealing with professional nurses. The emphasis on autonomy and decision-making participation conforms to those attributes usually associated with professionals and professional work. This supports, in part, the findings of other research on nurse collective bargaining, which maintains that issues related to the organization of nurses' jobs are at least as important as extrinsic rewards received.

The findings of these collective bargaining studies are important because they suggest that professional and organizational issues, such as autonomy and coordination and communication, are salient concerns among nurses in hospitals. Such evidence disputes the popular notions that salaries and other extrinsic rewards are the primary job concerns of the nurses. Further, collective bargaining research suggests that nursing staff and management may differ in their perceptions of issues and problems facing nursing. Because such differences imply administrative practices inconsistent with effective human resources management, a clearer understanding of nurses' role expectations in the hospital organization is warranted.

Nurses' Role in Hospitals—Process and Structure

The previous section surveyed the literature on two symptoms relevant to nurses and hospitals—turnover and collective bargaining. This research suggests that determinants of these outcomes may, in part, originate in the organizational structure and administrative practices of the hospital. The following section develops this discussion by focusing on four specific areas pertaining to the nurse's role in the hospital organization. It examines selectively the organizational conditions and processes that affect the role and functioning of hospital staff nurses in order to develop a comprehensive model of nursing outcomes. The topics addressed include: professional-bureaucratic conflict; transition from nursing student to hospital employee; nurse-management relations and nursing reorganization in hospitals.

Professional-Bureaucratic Role Conflict

The conflict between the hospital organization and its professional staff is a recurring theme in the literature on hospitals. Given the importance of autonomy and professional recognition as determinants of turnover and collective bargaining among nurses, the properties of the professional-hospital interface are worthy of review.

The early literature contrasting professional and bureaucratic organizations emphasized their inherently conflicting bases of control and authority. On the one hand, professionals draw on their expertise for authority and on collegial sanctioning for control. Bureaucracy, on the other hand, emphasizes an organizational position as the basis for authority and the principal of hierarchy, rules and regulations for control.

Scott (1966) maintains that such differences suggest two models for the organization of work. The professional model stipulates that each worker be provided with the range of skills required for performing the work as well as the norms directing standards of performance. The bureaucratic model prescribes dividing a task into a series of constituent activities. Each worker is then trained to perform a subset of those activities. According to Scott, the two models imply distinct areas of conflict and accommodation whenever an interface between them occurs, including rules governing organizational behavior, standards of performance, methods of supervision and identity with the organization or the profession.

The literature extensively treats the conflict engendered by the two contrasting systems (Scott 1965, Blau and Scott 1962, Hall 1967, 1969, Goss 1961, Engel 1970, Engel and Hall 1973, Sorensen and Sorensen 1974). These and other studies have attempted to document the incompatibility of bureaucratic and professional models of work by examining professionals in bureaucratic settings.

Blau and Scott (1962) maintain, on the basis of a review of the literature, that conflicts created by the interface of profession and bureaucracy are resolved by the bureaucratized professional in one of two ways. Some retain their identification with their professional group, are highly committed to their professional skills and look to professional colleagues for social support.

Others have less commitment to their specialized skills and come to identify with the program and procedures of their employing organization. The organizational conditions under which the two forms of conflict resolutions occur have only sporadically been examined in the literature.

Work in this area has yielded findings that challenge the notion that professions and bureaucracy are inherently conflicting systems (Meyer 1968, Kornhauser 1962, Engel 1970, Starkweather 1970, Coser 1958). The notion that bureaucracy and professionalism interact in non-linear fashion finds support in Engel's study of physicians in organizational settings (Engel 1970). She discovered that physicians working in moderately bureaucratic situations perceived themselves as having more autonomy than physicians working in either low or high bureaucratic settings. These findings suggest that the degree of bureaucratization, rather than its presence or absence, affects individual professionalism. Although not elaborated in the study, Engel's findings may also suggest that dimensions of bureaucracy, rather than bureaucracy as a unified set of characteristics, are associated with individual professionalism.

In an investigation of hospital surgical units, Coser (1958) found that highly centralized units generally displayed low degrees of formalized procedure and hierarchical authority arrangements. She argued that the nature of the centralized decision-making process leads to greater collegial interaction on the staff level, increased emphasis on problem solving and less emphasis on rule maintenance. These findings support the notion that bureaucratic structure and professionalism may be consistent under certain conditions.

The studies cited above indicate that dimensions of bureaucracy and profession do not invariably conflict and that structures are more or less supportive of professional role orientation.

Several studies have suggested structural solutions to the problem of professional-bureaucratic conflict. Pearlin (1962) examined the relationship between subunit structure and alienation among nurses working in a large mental hospital. He found an association between alienation and conditions that minimized interaction between supervisors and subordinates, and conditions that discourage cooperative work arrangements or, conversely, encourage isolated task assignments. Pearlin concluded that considerable structural diversity is subsumed under the same organization and that some structural arrangements can be alienating while others act as a barrier against alienation.

Goss (1961) noted that conflict was reduced between physicians and hospital administration when medical staff organization includes: formal and advisory control structures, professional expertise in the administrative staff, and performance by administrators of professional as well as administrative functions.

The nursing literature contains numerous studies suggesting an association among nurses' role conceptions, role conflict and the work context of their hospital or patient care unit (see Kramer 1968, 1969, Benner and Kramer 1972, Corwin 1961, Harrington and Theis 1968, Thorner 1955, Elpern 1974, Corwin and Taves 1962).

On a general level, Kramer (1974) proposed that a principle form of conflict resolution and role modification among hospital nurses is "value capitulation." According to Kramer, this is the process whereby nurses adjust their original role orientation and professional values to become consistent with those of the work setting. Nurses who remain in a work setting come to believe, for example, that work-setting procedures and goals are more operational than their own previously held standards and that they result in the "best possible care for the largest number of people."

Attempts to determine how the hospital organization is responsible for this modification in nurse role conceptions have been limited largely to three categories of studies. The first explores variation in role conceptions by hospital type (Pankratz and Pankratz 1974, Alutto 1971). Pankratz and Pankratz, for example, found that nurses in specialized or teaching hospitals maintained stronger professional orientations than nurses in community hospitals.

Alutto (1971) provided evidence that nurses in three hospital types clearly differed in their perceptions of and preferences for the source of influence in determining role orientations. Nurses in county hospitals, for example, saw their roles as determined by head nurses (bureaucratic), while those in community hospitals saw their roles as patient-defined (professional).

A second group of studies argued that a nurse's tenure and position in the hospital hierarchy influence her/his perception of organizational roles (Halberstein and Christ 1955, Marram 1971, Corwin and Taves 1962, Kramer 1969). For example, Halberstein and Christ demonstrated that head nurses and nursing directors perceived the nursing role as more autonomous than did staff nurses.

A third area of research has compared types of unit or staffing arrangements to determine their impact on nurse role conceptions (Harrington and Theis 1968, Elpern 1977, Benner and Kramer 1972, Holland 1973). Benner and Kramer (1972) compared the role orientations of nurses in special care units (SCU) to those of nurses in regular units. They argued that SCU nurses, by virtue of their work arrangements, would exhibit both strong professional and strong bureaucratic role orientations. Among those characteristics thought to promote professionalism in SCUs were high nurse-patient ratio, small number of patients, case assignment of patients, and frequent collegial contact. Factors supporting a bureaucratic orientation were technical orientation of the work and evaluation based on the efficient performance of technical tasks. Although no significant differences were found, the authors concluded that the co-presence of bureaucratic and professional work arrangements in SCUs served to increase role conflict and subsequently selected out nurses unable to accommodate the dualistic nature of their work environment.

Marram (1971) offered evidence that primary care unit nurses engaged in low task differentiation exhibited stronger professional attitudes than nurses in units practicing greater task differentiation. Based on cross-sectional comparisons, she further discovered that nurses in primary units retained their professional orientations while similar orientations among nurses in more differentiated units were gradually lost.

Harrington and Theis (1968) compared perceptions of baccalaureate nurses in three structurally disparate patient care units. Two of these units were characterized as traditional bureaucratic wards while the third was seen as innovative and non-bureaucratic. Nurses in the less bureaucratized unit expressed attitudes that structural features of the unit contributed positively to the fulfillment of the professional nursing function. Nurses in the more bureaucratized units felt that the same structural features acted as deterrents to professional nursing activity. Among the structural characteristics cited were work assignments, expectations of unit supervisors, communications, and staffing patterns and policies.

Although these and other works stress organizational accommodation to alleviate the professional-bureaucratic role conflict, few actually specify the process of organizational accommodation in longitudinal fashion. The cross-sectional relationships between structural characteristics and professional conflict suggest only that variation in structural arrangements exists within hospitals and that such variation is associated with the degree of conflict expressed by individuals in those organizations. With few exceptions, it remains to be demonstrated that a modification in the structural features of hospitals will accommodate the needs of their professional employees.

Transition from Nursing Student to Hospital Employee

A related body of nursing literature focuses on the problems of transition from nursing student to hospital employee (Corwin 1961, Corwin and Taves 1962, Kramer 1968, 1969, 1970, Benner and Kramer 1972).

These studies deal with various aspects of nurses' identification with personal ideals and institutional goals and the conflicts that occur from their pursuit of these in the hospital environment. Underlying much of this work is the notion that the values, norms, and ideology imparted during a nurse's education are inconsistent with the reality encountered in hospital work. This "reality shock" is thought to result in disillusionment and role conflict, which in turn are posited to lead to either a departure from the conflict-producing situation or readjustment of both values and roles over time.

Kramer's studies (1968, 1969) suggest that baccalaureate nursing graduates experience a significant shift in values shortly following hospital employment. Graduating nurses who expressed a high evaluation of professional standards and a low opinion of bureaucratic norms manifested a significant decrease in the former and an increase in the latter after hospital employment.

Corwin (1961) also examined the role conflicts experienced by newly graduated nurses in the hospital setting. In a study of 25 registered and 71 student nurses he found that degree nurses attempted to hold simultaneously professional and bureaucratic principles following graduation. Corwin claims that holding such dual roles results in conflict for the holder of such roles. By contrast, those nurses trained in diploma programs experienced a decline in their professional role orientations after graduation, while maintaining their initially high bureaucratic orientations.

The consequences of role conflict and lack of role clarity for the nurse and hospital have received only limited scrutiny in the literature (Lyons 1970, Hurka 1974). Lyons, for example, examined the need for role clarity and its relationship to job satisfaction, tension and withdrawal among nurses. Using survey methods, he discovered that perceived clarity of roles by nurses was negatively related to voluntary turnover, propensity to leave the job and job tension, and was positively associated with job satisfaction. It should be noted that most of these relationships applied only to those nurses who perceived a high need for role clarity.

In sum, role theory suggests two major determinants of job satisfaction among nurses: the degree of role conflict and the degree of role ambiguity experienced in the hospital context. These related concepts are seen to result from the multiple and competing demands on the nurse in the hospital setting and the discontinuity of nurses' expectations regarding their role in the hospital. To the extent that these concepts are predictive of work-related outcomes (e.g., turnover), they may provide a useful framework for considering managerial interventions to preclude such outcomes. Creation of new nursing roles, organizational restructuring and improved career mobility channels represent a few of the potentially fruitful areas of investigation in this area.

Nurse-Management Relations

The literature on nurse collective bargaining suggests that issues nurses perceive as important may not be similarly perceived by hospital management. These differences may reflect fundamental disagreement between nurses and administration on the role and function of nursing in the hospital. Given the obvious influence of style of hospital management on the practice of nursing, such differences may lead to adverse organizational consequences, notably poor job satisfaction and high turnover among nurses. Explanations of these differing perceptions of the nursing function are considered below.

Bloom, et al (1980), Hobart (1976) and Kelly (1972) suggest that current management practices toward nursing reflect a movement by hospital administrators to adopt the management principles of product-oriented industries. Bloom et al (1980) argue that these styles of management may not be entirely appropriate to the governance of service industries, such as hospitals.

One such industrial management model, the traditional model of management, assumes that employees neither want nor can handle work requiring creativity, self-direction or self-control. Extrinsic rewards, such as salary, are considered more important than rewards inherent in the work itself. A second industry-based model of management emphasizes high morale and similarity of needs among employees. Under this model, management's role is to plan and implement while employees are assumed to willingly cooperate with their supervisors contingent upon fulfillment of their needs.

Both these management models discount the importance of intrinsic motivation for work and mechanisms geared toward improving decision making and efficiency on an organizationwide level. To the extent that nurses value greater self-control and decision-making autonomy, styles of management currently practiced in hospitals may not be consistent with these objectives.

Indeed, the literature on organizations suggests that a critical set of activities for professionals in complex organizations is the maintenance of autonomy through participation in organizational decision making. Such decision making is not totally unbounded but occurs within organizationally defined constraints (Alutto and Acito, 1974). In a study of 197 nurses in two urban hospitals, Alutto and Vredenburgh (1977) classified 75 percent of the sample as "decisionally deprived" in that their desired participation in decisions within the hospital exceeded actual participation. Among those areas in which participation was desired but not achieved were deciding how ancillary personnel would be used, planning and designing facilities for nursing care and determining how nursing practices would be performed. The data further suggested that nurses expressing decisional deprivation tended to be in less authoritative organizational positions, and were younger and less experienced than nurses experiencing equilibrium between decisional preferences and actions. Finally, individuals desiring more decision-making involvement experienced greater job tension and career dissatisfaction. Earlier studies (Alutto and Acito 1974) noted an association between degree of decision deprivation and levels of satisfaction with promotions, pay, work and supervision.

Scott et al (1972) suggest a more theoretical explanation for the difference in administrators' and nurses' views of the nursing role. They argue that perceptions of the technology of work are largely a function of the proximity of the perceiver to the core technology of the organization. Those who are relatively close to the production function (e.g., patient care) tend to be concerned with aspects of production that are highly uncertain and variable. To deal effectively with these uncertainties, these individuals aspire to organizational arrangements that allow autonomy and decision-making discretion. Administrators, being further removed from the production function, emphasize the uniform and predictable aspects of work. They choose organizational arrangements characterized by standardized procedures and a structured approach to production. The extent to which nurses and administrators conform to this theoretical model is likely to determine the difference in the perception of the nursing function between the two groups. This theory further predicts that the organizational power vested in hospital administrators results in administrative arrangements that reflect the task conceptions of the administrators rather than the nurse. Thus, much of the disaffection nurses display toward hospital nursing may emanate from the manner in which their tasks are organized or the lack of autonomy with which they must approach their work.

Indirect support for this argument is provided by Alexander (1982). In a study of 730 registered nurses in 142 patient care units, he found that considerable variation in work arrangements existed in patient care units within and among hospitals. Controlling for technological characteristics of the work, supervisory style of head nurses and individual attributes of the nurse, such variation was significantly associated with the professional role orientations of staff nurses. Unit size, unit autonomy and task coordination were particularly strong determinants of these role orientations.

Nursing Reorganization

In response to the organizational conflicts expressed by hospital nurses and the changing nature of patient care, a number of administrative changes have been initiated in selected hospital settings. As documented in the literature, those changes relevant to hospital nursing may be grouped into two categories: reorganization of nursing departments and expansion and redefinition of nursing roles.

In general, the literature on reorganization of hospital nursing has been nonempirical or descriptive in nature. What little empirical research exists suffers from the absence of clear conceptual frameworks, small sample sizes and reliance on perceptual, rather than objective, measures. Some of these problems may reflect a lack of widespread organizational change in hospitals and hospital nursing services. To the extent of insufficient data, examination their impact must be limited to isolated case studies and descriptive reports.

The literature on reorganization of nursing services in the hospital has concentrated largely on the decentralization of nursing services. An assumption underlying much of this work is that administrative decentralization is conducive to critical thinking, participatory decision making and individual autonomy, and that these will in turn reduce turnover, improve nursing morale and enhance patient care (Thomas 1969, Seday 1974, Fine 1977, and Nehls et al 1974). Unfortunately, the vast majority of the work in administrative change has not been empirically oriented. Neither qualitative nor quantitative evaluations of such administrative innovations have been performed in a coordinated and systematic fashion (Maas 1973). Instead, the thrust of the literature on decentralization has been to propose administrative mechanisms that would reduce bureaucratic ineffectiveness and, at the same time, enhance the professional role of the nurse (Simms 1973, Howe 1969, Mahowald 1974, and Starkweather 1970). Simms (1973), for example, argues that decentralized administrative arrangements allow nursing administration to engage in education and research functions while enabling staff nurses to direct their own efforts, thereby increasing responsibility and accountability for personal nursing care.

Fine (1977) posits that decentralized nursing is a necessary consequence of the increasing complexity of nursing tasks, the intensive technologies in many patient care units, and the unstable environments in which hospitals operate. Such conditions, argues Fine, necessitate lateral communication and cooperation between nurses and other groups in the hospital and enable nurses to develop self-regulation and participatory roles.

A major assumption underlying many of the efforts to reorganize nursing jobs has been that such reorganization will satisfy an inherent set of needs among nurses. This perspective asserts that people have needs, that jobs have objective characteristics and that job attitudes result from their interface. According to Salancik and Pfeffer (1978) and others, the needs satisfaction model fails to account for the social context of work as a factor that influences attitudes and behaviors of workers. Needs and attitudes, rather than being immutable attributes of the individual, are adapted to the social context and the information that context provides. This suggests that attitudes are a function of the individual's interpretation and perception of the work environment, not a result of social or organizational rewards satisfying personal needs. The literature indeed supports the social information processing perspective on job attitudes formation. Alexander (1982), Herman and Hulein (1972) and O'Reilly and Roberts (1972) compared individual and social structure effects on individual job attitudes and found that organizational characteristics explained job attitudes better than individual characteristics.

The programmatic implications of these alternative perspectives on job attitudes are profound. The needs-satisfaction approach has led to a focus design as a mechanism for realizing the inherently satisfying nature of work for meeting various human needs. Results achieved by job redesign, however, may emanate from a process of social cooptation rather than need satisfaction (Salancik and Pfeffer 1978). That is, individuals come to define their work situations and their job attitudes using criteria imposed by the organization and its managers. Positive job attitudes result from the salience of organizationally defined job characteristics and the expectations for change in those characteristics. Failure of job redesign efforts may not lie in the failure to meet workers needs, but in the failure to render certain job characteristics and their change salient to the worker. According to the social information processing perspective, workers possess the ability to construct satisfaction through their selective perceptions and interpretations of the social environment in which they work. The implication of this perspective is that, to the extent that problems are interpreted by the individual as being under his or her province or control, the individual will be more apt to take action to remedy these problems. Workers committed to and responsible for a situation are more likely to find satisfaction and meaning from it. Alternatively, the assumption of fixed needs and fixed work environment implies a lack of control by workers that usually produces alienation and job dissatisfaction.

Conclusions and Recommendations

The paucity of quality research on the organizational structure of hospital nursing does not lend itself well to administrative or policy decisions in nursing. To date, the best research on nursing has produced only sets of loosely related, empirical determinants of outcomes (e.g., job satisfaction, professionalism, turnover). Poor methodology and inadequate conceptualization are the major limitations in most nursing-related studies. These defects preclude efforts to systematically relate the numerous investigations in the areas and develop cumulative knowledge on nursing issues. However, on the positive side, the quality of research on nursing is improving noticeably and existing research provides a wealth of descriptive material from which more substantial conceptual frameworks may be developed. Pending further upgrading of nursing research, other more established areas of investigation might shed considerable light on nursing problems. For example, industrial relations, sociology, social-psychology, psychology and organizational behavior may contain research findings and conceptual frameworks appropriate to hospital nursing.

Despite the limitations of much of related research, several tentative conclusions emerge from the literature.

1. The literature suggests that much of the conflict nurses experience in the hospital setting may be attributed to their multiple roles in the hospital organization. Essentially, nurses must walk an organizational tightrope between three disparate hospital constituencies. As independent professionals, nurses are responsible for providing professional nursing care for the patients under their charge. They are, at the same time, agents of physicians in carrying out physician orders for treatment. Also nurses are members of the hospital organization and must involve themselves with the day-to-day administration of the patient care unit. Nurses must balance their own professional standards with individual physician's orders for the care of individual patients and the need to manage an aggregate of cases in an administratively acceptable manner (Freidson 1970). As these demands are often contradictory, nurses are subject to role conflict or role ambiguity, which are thought to relate to adverse organizational consequences, such as job satisfaction,

alienation and ultimately turnover and collective bargaining.

2. The emphasis in the literature on participatory decision making by nurses suggests that management policies related to nursing be initiated bilaterally in order to be effective. That is, nurses must fully participate in the planning and implementation of these policies if they are to be consistent with the model of management of professionals. Further, administrative changes aimed at reducing nurse role conflict and clarifying role definition in the hospital will not be effective unless nurses themselves actively participate in designing and implementing them. Innovations emanating from hospital or nursing administration without the collaboration of nursing staff run the risk of being construed no differently than other centralized administrative mandates.

3. Recent research on hospital organizations (Alexander 1982, Comstock 1975, Comstock and Scott 1977) has produced evidence that considerable structural and technological variation may occur within as well as among hospitals. A major bias of much of the literature relating to hospital nursing is the tendency to discount such intraorganizational variation. It assumes that all hospitals are equivalent in terms of the organizational conditions under which nurses work. The danger in this assumption becomes acute if policy recommendations engendered by hospital-level research are inappropriate for the diverse array of organizational and technological conditions within those organizations. For example, a managerial practice which benefits nurses in medical or surgical units may not be suitable for intensive care unit nurses. It is important, therefore, to pursue research that specifies the varying conditions under which nurses practice in hospitals and the extent to which such variation is associated with outcomes relevant to nursing retention.

4. The literature suggests that role conflict, job dissatisfaction and professional alienation among nurses occur most frequently among newly graduated registered nurses, especially those holding baccalaureate degrees. A recurring thesis in this literature is that these adverse outcomes on nursing result in part from the incompatability of values and expectations inculcated during nursing education and the operational realities encountered in the hospital. However, further investigation is needed on the relationship between elements of nursing education and the work environment of hospitals and the extent to which modifications in hospital work arrangements affect nonnursing operations in the hospital.

5. The numerous experiments in reorganization of organizational structures for nursing have met with only partial success in alleviating nursing problems in hospitals. This does not imply, however, that such innovations are inherently ineffective. One explanation for the potential failure of these innovations has been previously cited as the unilateral manner in which they are implemented. Equally important is the absence of rigorous evaluation of these administrative practices. Without such evaluation it becomes difficult to specify the benefits and costs that accrue to a hospital adopting a new system of nursing organization and the conditions under which a particular organizational practice will function effectively. Lack of sound evaluation has allowed nursing innovations to become normative catchwords (e.g., primary nursing, team nursing, joint practice), the substance of which varies greatly from hospital to hospital. Success or failure of the innovation, therefore, is likely to be just as varied. To avoid this situation, evaluation mechanisms are

needed that allow examination not only of the outcomes of the administrative intervention but also of the theoretical foundations on which administrative changes are based.

Preliminary Model of Hospital Nursing Outcomes

Based on findings from the existing descriptive and analytic literature, a preliminary model of organizational outcomes related to nursing can be proposed. The model is not sufficiently developed to yield predictions regarding the relationship between specific dimensions of hospital structure and intermediate and long-range nursing outcomes. It is intended to serve only as a general framework for generating research questions and to act as a tool for considering potential interrelationships among variables affecting organizational outcomes relevant to nursing.

The model departs from previous research in two major respects. First, it is comprehensive in scope, addressing multiple causes of outcomes on nursing in hospitals and their interrelationships. Previous research, with several notable exceptions, has focused largely on single outcomes and univariate determinants of those outcomes. Second, the model proposes the theoretical processes that result in particular outcomes on nursing. Much of the research on nursing to date has examined only the empirical determinants of nursing-related outcomes.

The proposed model stipulates that structural factors inherent in the hospital work environment represent the primary determinants of the nurses' role in the hospital setting and the properties attendant to that role (e.g., autonomy). These properties will, in turn, bear directly on a degree of role and organizational conflict experienced by the nurse as well as heighten the degree of job satisfaction. A major assumption in the model is that individual attributes of the nurse, such as professional socializations and marital status, act as mediating variables in the structure-role relationship. For example, the model might predict that the effects of job differentiation on perceptions of autonomy are mediated by the type of education the nurse has received and the amount of experience she has had in a particular hospital unit.

Clearly, development and refinement of the proposed model will require a systematic program of investigation that includes:

- empirical specification of the relationship of structural variables at the individual, unit and hospital levels (the work of Comstock and Scott 1977, Scott and Flood 1978 should provide a strong foundation for such research);
- analysis of the relationship between hospital organization and specific dimensions of nursing role structure, including the extent to which individual attributes of the nurse mediate such relationships; and
- determination of the elements of the nurse's role which best predict the extent of role conflict and satisfaction in the hospital settings. Because relatively little empirical research has been performed in this area, it may behoove investigators to approach the task incrementally. When empiri-

cal evidence is sufficient, a more comprehensive treatment of the model may be attempted.

Hospital Organizational Structure	Personal Attributes	Nursing Role Structure	Nursing Outcomes	Organizational Outcomes
Job Content (Individual Level)	**Professional Socialization**	**Job autonomy**	**Job satisfaction**	**Turnover**
1. Differentiation	1. Type of RN degree	**Decision making participation**	**Role conflict**	**Collective bargaining**
2. Standardization	2. Highest degree achieved		**Alienation**	
3. Rotation		**Professional-relations**		
4. Rewards		**Role identification**		
5. Patient care technology	**Organizational/ Occupational Tenure**			
	1. Years in unit			
Job Context (Unit Level)	2. Years in hospital			
1. Coordination—vertical	3. Years in nursing			
2. Coordination—lateral				
3. Unit autonomy	**Socio-Demographic Variables**			
4. Size of unit				
5. Evaluation structure	1. Age			
6. Mobility structure	2. Marital status			
7. Centralization	3. Number and age of children			
	4. Occupation of spouse			
Hospital Context (Organizational Level)				
1. Teaching institution				
2. Hospital size				
3. Urban/rural				
4. Centralization				

Bibliography

Alexander, J. *The Organizational Structure of Hospital Nursing Units: Its Effect on Staff Professionalism.* Ann Arbor: UMI Press, 1982.

Alutto, J. Variation in hospital employment and influence perceptions among nursing personnel. *Journal of Health and Social Behavior* 12:30, Mar. 1971.

Alutto, J. and Acito, F. Decisional participation by and sources of satisfaction: A study of manufacturing personnel. *Academy of Management Journal* 17:160, Mar. 1974.

Alutto, J. and Balasco, J.A. Typology for participation in organizational decision making. *Administrative Science Quarterly* 17:117, Mar. 1972.

Alutto, J. and Vredenburgh, D. Characteristics of decisional participation by nurses. *Academy of Management Journal* 20:341, June 1977.

Behling, O.C. and Kosmo, R. Reducing nursing turnover: Job satisfaction not the only cause. *Hospitals* 45:124, Feb. 1, 1971.

Benner, P. and Kramer, M. Role conceptions and integrated behavior of nurses in special care and regular hospital nursing units. *Nursing Research* 21:20, Jan.–Feb. 1972.

Benton, D.A. and White, H.C. Satisfaction of job factors for registered nurses. *Journal of Nursing Administration* 2:55, Nov.–Dec. 1972.

Blau, P. and Scott, W.R. *Formal Organizations,* p. 60. San Francisco: Chandler Publishing Co., 1962.

Bloom, J.R., Parlette, G.N. and O'Reilly, C.A. Collective bargaining by nurses: A comparative analysis of management and employee perceptions. *Health Care Management Review* 5:25, Winter 1980.

Brief, A.P. Turnover among hospital nurses: A suggested model. *Journal of Nursing Administration* 6:55, Oct. 1976.

Brief et al. Anticipatory socialization and role stress among registered nurses. *Journal of Health and Social Behavior* 20:161, June 1979.

Bullough, B. Is the nurse practitioner role a service of increased work satisfaction? *Nursing Research* 23:14, Jan.–Feb. 1974.

Burlington, T., Lentz, E. and Wilson, R.N. *The Give and Take in Hospitals: A Study of Human Organization in Hospitals.* New York: Putnam, 1956.

Campbell, D. and Stanley, J. *Experimental and Quasi-experimental Design for Research.* Chicago: Rand McNally, 1963.

Comstock, D. Technology and Context: A Study of Hospital Patient Care Units. Unpublished dissertation. Stanford University, 1975.

Comstock, D. and Scott, W.R. Technology and the structure of subunits: Distinguishing individual and workgroup effects. *Administrative Science Quarterly,* 22:177, June 1977.

Corwin, R. The professional employee: A study in the conflict of nursing roles. *American Journal of Sociology* 66:604, May 1961.

Corwin, R. and Taves, M. Some concommitants of bureaucratic and professional conceptions of the nurse role. *Nursing Research* 11:223, Fall 1962.

Coser, R. Authority and decision making in a hospital: A comparative analysis. *American Sociological Review* 23:56, Feb. 1958.

Dauw, D. Human factors outrank salary as turnover cause in this hospital. *Hospital Topics* 44:65, Aug. 1966.

Diamond, L.K. and Fox, D.J. Turnover among hospital staff nurses. *Nursing Outlook* 6:388, July 1958.

Elpern, E. Structural and organizational support for primary nursing. *Nursing Clinic of North America* 12:205, June 1977.

Engel, G. Professional autonomy and bureaucratic organization. *Administrative Science Quarterly* 15:12, Mar. 1970.

Engel, G. and Hall, R. The growing industrialization of the professions. In Freidson, E. (comp.) *The Professions and Their Prospects.* Beverly Hills, CA: Sage Publications, 1973.

Everly II, G.S. and Falcione, R.L. Perceived dimensions of job satisfaction for staff registered nurses. *Nursing Research* 25:346, Sept.–Oct. 1976.

Federation of American Hospitals. The nurse shortage: A national dilemma. *Review* 13:12, Apr.–May 1980.

Fine, R. Decentralization and staffing. *Nursing Administration Quarterly* 1:59, 1977.

Fralic, M.F. Nursing shortage: Coping today and planning for tomorrow. *Hospitals* 54:65, May 1, 1980.

Freidson, E. *The Profession of Medicine.* New York: Dodd, Mead & Co., Inc., 1970.

Goss, M. Influence and authority among physicians in an outpatient clinic. *American Sociological Review* 26:39, Feb. 1961.

Grand, N.L. Nursing ideologies and collective bargaining. *Journal of Nursing Administration* 3:29, Mar.–Apr. 1973.

Halberstein, R. and Christ, E. *Professionalizer, Traditionalizer and Utilizer: An Interpretive Study of the Work of the General Duty Nurse in Non-metropolitan Central Missouri General Hospitals.* Columbia, MO: University of Missouri, 1955.

Hall, R. Some organizational considerations in professional-bureaucratic relationships. *Administrative Science Quarterly* 12:461, Dec. 1967.

_________. Professionalization and bureaucratization. *American Sociological Review* 33:92, Feb. 1969.

Harrington, H. and Theis, C. Institutional factors received by baccalaureate graduates as influencing their performance as staff nurses. *Nursing Research* 17:228, 1968.

Hobart, C. Collective bargaining with professionals: Conflict, containment or accommodation? *Health Care Management Review* 1:7, Spring 1976.

Herman, J. and Hulein, C. Studying organizational attitudes from individual and organizational frames of reference. *Organizational Behavior and Human Performance* 8:84, 1972.

Holland, T. Organizational structure and institutional care. *Journal of Health and Social Behavior* 14:241, Sept. 1973.

Howe, E.G. Decentralization aids coordination of patient care services. *Hospitals* 43:53, Mar. 1, 1969.

Hurka, S.J. Organizational environment and work satisfaction. *Dimensions in Health Service* 51:41, Jan. 1974.

Jelinek, R. and Dennis, L. *A Review and Evaluation of Nursing Productivity.* DHEW Publication no. (HRA) 77–15. Washington, D.C.: U.S. Government Printing Office, 1976.

Kase, S.J. and Swenson, B. Costs of hospital-sponsored orientation and inservice education for registered nurses. *Health Manpower References.* DHEW Publication no. (HRA) 77–25. Washington, D.C.: U.S. Government Printing Office, 1976.

Kelly, D. Neither malice nor conspiracy. *Supervisor Nurse* 3:8, Apr. 1972.

Knopf, L. *RN's One and Five Years After Graduation.* New York: National League for Nursing, 1975.

Kornhauser, W. *Scientists in Industry.* Berkeley: University of California Press, 1962.

Kramer, M. Role models, role conceptions, and role deprivation. *Nursing Research* 17:115, Mar.–Apr. 1968.

_________. Collegiate graduate nurses in medical center hospitals: Mutual challenge or duel. *Nursing Research* 18:196, May–June 1969.

_________. Role conceptions of baccalaureate nurses and success in hospital nursing. *Nursing Research* 19:428, Sept.–Oct. 1970.

_________. Team nursing—A means or an end? *Nursing Outlook* 19:648, Oct. 1971.

_________. *Reality Shock: Why Nurses Leave Nursing.* St. Louis, MO: C.V. Mosby, 1974.

Kramer, M. and Baker, C. Nursing exodus: Can we prevent it? *Journal of Nursing Administration* 1:15, May–June 1971.

Kravit, S. Collective bargaining for professionals. *Supervisor Nurse* 40:46, July 1973.

Levine, E. Nursing supply and requirements: The current status and future prospects. In Millman, M.L. (ed.), *Nursing Personnel and the Changing Health Care System*. Cambridge, MA: Ballinger Publishing Co., 1978.

Lyons, T. Reducing nursing turnover: An approach. *Hospitals* 44:74, Oct. 16, 1970.

Maas, M. Nurse autonomy and accountability in organized nursing services. *Nursing Forum* 12:237, 1973.

Mahowald, J., Freeman, J. and Dietsche, B. Decentralization of nursing authority. *Supervisor Nurse* 5:40, Mar. 1974.

Maritz, D. Management principles and nursing: The inefficiency of efficiency. *Supervisor Nurse* 11:40, Mar. 1980.

Marlow, H.L. The registered nurse and employee needs. *Nursing Outlook* 14:62, Nov. 1966.

Marram, G. Visibility of Work and the Evaluation Process: Evaluation and Authority for Nurses in Hospitals and Teachers in Open and Closed Schools. Unpublished doctoral dissertation. Stanford University, 1971.

McCloskey, J. Influence of rewards and incentives on staff nurse turnover rate. *Nursing Research* 23:239, May–June 1974.

McClure, M.C. The Reasons for Hospital Staff Nurse Resignations. Unpublished dissertation. Columbia University, 1972.

Meyer, M. Expertness and the span of control. *American Sociological Review* 33:944, Dec. 1968.

Munson, F.C. and Heda, S.S. An instrument for measuring satisfaction. *Nursing Research* 23:159, Mar.–Apr. 1974.

Nehls et al. Planned change: A quest for nursing autonomy. *Journal of Nursing Administration* 4:23, Jan.–Feb. 1974.

O'Reilly, C. and Roberts, K. Individual differences in personality, position in the organization and job satisfaction. *Organizational Behavior and Human Performance* 14:144, 1972.

Pankratz, L. and Pankratz, D. Nursing autonomy and patients' rights: Development of a nursing attitude scale. *Journal of Health and Social Behavior* 15:211, Sept. 1975.

Pearlin, L.I. Alienation from work: A study of nursing personnel. *American Sociological Review*, 27:314, June 1962.

Price, J. *Handbook of Organizational Measurement*, pp. 175, 177, 179, Lexington, MA: D.C. Heath and Co., 1972.

Price J. and Mueller, C. A causal model for turnover for nurses. *Academy of Management Journal* 24:543, Sept. 1981.

Revans, R.W. *Standards for Morale: Cause and Effect in Hospitals*. London: Oxford University Press, 1964.

Roth, A., Graham, D. and Schmittling, G. *1977 National Sample of Registered Nurses: A Report on the Nurse Population and Factors Affecting Their Supply*. Dept. of Commerce, Publication no. HRP-0900603. Washington, D.C.: U.S. Government Printing Office.

Salancik, G. and Pfeffer, J. A social information processing approach to job attitudes and task design. *Administrative Science Quarterly* 23:224, June 1978.

Saleh, S.D., Lee, R.J. and Prien, E.P. Why nurses leave their jobs—An analysis of female turnover. *Personnel Administration* 28:25, Jan.–Feb. 1965.

Scott, W.R. Reactions to supervision in heteronomous professional organizations. *Administrative Science Quarterly* 10:65, 1965.

________. Professional in Bureaucracies—Areas of Conflict. In Vollmer, H. and Mills, D. (eds.), *Professionalization*, pp, 265–275. Englewood Cliffs, NJ: Prentice Hall, 1966.

Scott et al. Task Conceptions and Work Arrangements. Standard Center for Research and Development in Teaching. Memo. no. 97, 1972.

Seday, A.J. Developing nurses' ability to manage: The roles of trust, participation and commitment. *Journal of Continuing Education in Nursing* 5:7, Jan.–Feb., 1974.

Seybolt, J.W., Pavett, C. and Walker, D.D. Turnover among nurses: It can be managed. *Journal of Nursing Administration* 8:4, Sept. 1978.

Simms, L.L. Administrative changes and implications for nursing practice in the hospital. *Nursing Clinics of North America* 8:227, June 1973.

Sloan, F.A. The Geographic Distribution of Nurses and Public Policy. Health Manpower References. DHEW Publication no. (HRA) 75–53. Washington, D.C.: U.S. Government Printing Office, 1975.

Sorenson, J. and Sorenson, T. The conflict of professionals in bureaucratic organizations. *Administrative Science Quarterly* 19:98, 1974.

Starkweather, D. Rationale for decentralization in large hospitals. *Hospital Administration*: 15:27, Spring 1970.

________. Hospital organizational, performance and size. *Inquiry* 10:10, Sept. 1973.

Stickler, K.B. and Velghe, J.C. Why nurses form unions. *Hospital Forum* 23:14, Mar. 1980.

Thomas, L.A. A rationale for nursing administration. *American Journal of Nursing* 69:774, Apr. 1969.

Thorner, J. Nursing: The fundamental significance of an institutional pattern. *American Sociological Review* 20:531, Oct. 1955.

U.S. Veteran's Administration. *Survey of Factors Relating to Job Satisfaction Among VA Nurses 1960–1970.* Washington, D.C.: U.S. Government Printing Office, 1973.

Weisman, C., Alexander, C. and Chase, G. Job satisfaction among hospital nurses: A longitudinal analysis. *Health Services Research* 15:341, Winter 1980.

White, C.H. and Maguire, M.C. Job satisfaction and dissatisfaction among hospital nursing supervisors: The applicability of Herzberg's theory. *Nursing Research* 22:25, Jan.–Feb. 1973.

Appendixes

Appendix 1

SURVEY OF CORPORATE NURSING IN MULTIHOSPITAL SYSTEMS

The emergence of multihospital systems is purported to influence health care delivery. Literature dealing with multihospital systems emphasizes their advantages in capital formation, economy of scale benefits accrued by larger systems, shared expertise and others. Little has been written about how multihospital systems have or will affect nursing in member hospitals or about how nursing will affect the developing organizational modes of these systems. Lack of information about these possible influences and frequent reference to the impact of multihospital systems on nursing led to an invitational conference attended by nurses from multihospital system corporations and, eventually, to this survey.

METHODOLOGY

The survey instrument used in this study was developed from the proceedings of an invitational conference held to explore features of corporate nursing in multihospital systems that affect nursing in member hospitals. Fifteen nurses, either holding positions with direct responsibility for nursing at the corporate level in multihospital systems or representing the multihospital system, attended the conference. A summary of the conference proceedings was sent to the participants for review and comment and was revised accordingly.

Content from the conference proceedings was used to develop the survey instrument, which was sent to selected participants for validation. The survey instrument was then refined.

To identify persons at the corporate level with direct responsibility for nursing, postcards were sent to the 256 multihospital systems listed in the *Directory of Multihospital Systems, 1981*.[1] Surveys were sent to all persons listed from the 178 returned postcards. A total of 47 completed and usable surveys were analyzed for this

---

[1]American Hospital Association. *Directory of Multihospital Systems*. Chicago: American Hospital Association, 1983.

report. A number of the systems contacted called and indicated that the survey did not apply to them, but no record was kept of the number of calls received.

Description of the Sample

Multihospital systems that returned the survey were compared with those listed in the *Directory of Multihospital Systems, 1982*. Of the 47 total returns, 40 were from listed multihospital systems, three were not listed and four were not identified. The seven unlisted systems had a total of 61 hospitals, and the entire sample had 900 hospitals.

Respondents listed in the directory were compared with the total directory listings to evaluate the proportion of hospitals and beds represented in the survey sample. The comparison by type of organizational control and size is shown in Table 1a.

Table 1a

Number and percentages of respondents listed in the *Directory of Multihospital Systems, 1982*, listed by type of multihospital system organizational control and number of hospitals and beds.

Type of Organizational Control	Multihospital System: Total Systems Listed	Respondents: Number	Respondents: % of Total
Catholic church related	104	9	[09]
Other church related	21	10	[48]
Not-for-profit	104	12	[12]
Total not-for-profit	[229]	[31]	[14]
Investor owned	27	9	[33]
Total systems	[256]	[40]	[16]
Number of hospitals	1,924	839	[44]
Number of beds	359,618	129,453	[36]

Table 1b shows the number of hospitals in the reporting multihospital systems.

Respondents represented all categories of organizational control used in the *Directory of Multihospital Systems, 1982;* 16 percent of the total number of multihospital systems listed, 44 percent of the hospitals and 36 percent of the beds. Twenty of the respondents were from multihospitals that had both owned, leased or sponsored hospitals and contract-managed hospitals. The number of hospitals per system ranged from 7 to 340. Four respondents were from multihospital systems with only contract-managed hospitals and 17 were from system that only owned, leased or sponsored hospitals. Of these 17 systems, 12 were not-for-profit with seven or fewer hospitals and four were investor-owned with 11 to 87 hospitals. The number of hospitals ranged between two and 87. In the total sample, seven percent of the hospitals had nurse unions (63 of 900). The survey questions did not differentiate the number of unions for registered nurses; the data represent only the number of hospitals with unions.

Data were examined according to type of multihospital system, organizational control and size; but no discernable patterns were found. Data were categorized

Table 1b

Number of hospitals per system in the sample.

	Total		Centralized				Decentralized			
			NCL		NNCL		NCL		NNCL	
# Hospitals	#	%	#	%	#	%	#	%	#	%
Range										
1–4	15	32	0	0	2	200	3	20	11	42
5–9	9	19	1	20	–	–	2	13	6	23
10–14	7	15	0	0	–	–	4	27	3	12
15–19	2	4	1	20	–	–	0	0	1	4
20+	13	28	3	60	–	–	6	40	4	15
# with unionized hospitals	11	23	1	20	–	–	4	27	6	23
No answer	1	2	0	0	–	–			1	4
TOTAL HOSPITALS	900	100								

according to an organizational perspective of centralized or decentralized multihospital systems. In each category, subcategories of a nurse employed at the corporate level (NCL) or no nurse employed at the corporate level (NNCL) were used. Throughout the report, "NCL" refers to nurse at the corporate level with designated responsibility for nursing and "NNCL" refers to no nurse employed at the corporate level in this capacity. Table 2 provides the number of respondents in each category. In the total sample, 43 percent of the respondents had one or more NCLs.

Table 2

Number of multihospital systems employing a nurse at the corporate level in a position with responsibility for nursing according to type of position.

	Types of Organization		
Corporate Level Position For Nursing	**Centralized**	**Decentralized**	**Total**
Yes	5 [11%]	15 [32%]	[N=20] 43%
No	1 [2%]	26 [55%]	[N=27] 57%
TOTAL	6 [13%]	41 [87%]	[N=47] 100%

FINDINGS

The majority of the 47 systems responding were decentralized; of these, 32 percent employed an NCL. All except one of the centralized systems employed an NCL.

Ninety-five percent of the systems that employed an NCL had only one or two positions. One system reported more than two positions (35 percent); 12 reported one position (60 percent); and seven reported two positions (5 percent).

Titles of Corporate-level Nursing Positions

Titles of NCLs were grouped according to position. The most frequently reported title was vice president (28 percent). The four most frequently used titles are shown in Table 3. In many instances, the title included either "nurse" or "patient services," such as "vice president, patient services."

Table 3

Distribution of corporate-level nursing position titles in reporting multihospital systems.

Title	Number of Multihospital Systems
Vice President	11
Consultant	8
Director	6
Assistant Director	3
Other (contains one system with 14 titles)	10

Date Position Was Initiated

The earliest date of initiation reported for the corporate nurse position was 1976. Twenty of the 24 positions for which dates of initiation were reported were initiated in 1979 or later. The year the corporate nurse position was initiated is shown in Table 4 for the 20 systems that reported information about date of initiation.

Table 4

Year corporate-level position with responsibility for nursing was initiated.

	Multihospital System		
Year	Centralized* [N=5]	Decentralized* [N=15]	Total 20
1976	1	1	2
1977	1	1	2
1978	–	–	0
1979	3	2	5
1980	1	6	7
1981	1	4	5
1982	–	2	2
1983	–	1	1
	7	17	24

*Eight systems listing more than one position.

Corporate Functions Related to Nursing in Member Hospitals

Respondents were asked to list corporate functions related to nursing in member hospitals. A total of 17 functions were reported; nine of these were reported by 22 percent or more respondents. The percentage of systems reporting each of the nine functions is shown in Table 5.

Table 5

Percentages of corporate functions relating to nursing in member hospitals by type of organization and NCL.

	Multihospital System					
Function	**Total** %	**N=6 Total Centralized** %	**N=41 Total Decentralized** %	**N=20 With NCL** %	**N=27 With NNCL** %	**% Functions Provided by Other Dept. or Division**
Management Education	62	67	55	95	41	30
Consultation	62	83	59	200	33	13
Staff Nurse Recruitment	62	83	34	70	19	19
Personnel Comp. and Benefit	55	67	54	70	44	40
Nursing Dept. Policy	49	67	46	85	70	11
Quality Assurance	47	67	38	75	67	23
Risk Management	45	50	38	70	67	23
Search & Selection for DON	10	83	49	85	74	9
Research	10	50	17	45	4	11

Other functions listed by nine respondents were trustee education (N=2); medical staff organization (N=2); contracts with schools (N=2); contracts with nurse registries (N=2); network sharing and support for directors of nursing (N=2); continuing education (N=2); infection control (N=1); and hospitalwide licensure (N=1).

Of the nine most frequently reported functions, management education and consultation were most consistently reported, followed by director of nursing search and selection, nursing department policy, quality assurance and risk management. Personnel compensation and benefit functions were most frequently provided by a corporate department or division other than nursing. In most cases, both nursing and other departments were listed as providing the function. Functions provided on an advisory basis or on request only are shown in Table 7.

Table 7

Percentages of functions provided on advisory or request only basis by type of organization and corporate nurse.*

				Multihospital System							
Function	**N=47 Total With Function**	**N=47 Total With Advisory**	**N=47 Total With Request**	**N=5 Centralized With NCL**		**N=15 Decentralized With NCL**		**N=20 Total With NCL**		**N=26 Decentralized With NNCL**	
Management Education	62	23	28	20	40	40	53	35	35	15	23
Consultation	62	32	40	40	40	47	67	45	60	23	27
Staff Nurse Recruitment	62	17	28	40	60	27	27	30	35	8	23
Personnel Comp. and Benefit	55	19	15	40	40	40	60	25	15	12	19
Nursing Dept. Policy	49	30	30	60	60	33	53	40	55	23	12
Quality Assurance	47	32	28	60	60	40	40	45	45	23	15
Risk Management	45	21	15	40	40	20	20	25	25	19	8
Search & Selection for DON	10	23	36	20	60	40	60	40	60	12	19
Research	10	9	11	10	40	20	13	20	20	0	4

*The one centralized system with NNCL was not included in this table.

Nursing Advisory Committees

Nursing advisory committees were reported by 32 percent of the decentralized systems. Of these, 15 percent reported ad hoc committees and 17 percent reported appointed committees. Of the total systems, 15 percent of the systems with an advisory committee for nursing were centrally located and seven percent were regionally located.

Corporate Committees with Nurse Membership

The number of corporate committees with nurse membership reported was greatest in decentralized systems with a NCL. Table 8 indicates the number of committees reported by respondents.

Member Hospital Relationships between the Corporate Level and Nursing

Respondents were asked to describe how the corporation related to nursing in member hospitals. Of the 47 respondents, 49 percent indicated that nursing in member hospitals related to the corporation through corporate headquarters. This group included all except one system that reported having a NCL. Table 9 shows the types of relationships reported by the 34 systems for which the information was given and the channel for communication given by respondents.

Table 8

Number of corporate committees with nurse membership by type of organization and corporate nurse.

Number of Committees	Multihospital System: Centralized NCL	Decentralized NCL	Decentralized NNCL
One	–	1	4
Two	–	4	2
Three	1	1	4
Four	2	3	2
Five or more	–	2	2
Total systems with committees	3 (50%)	11 (73%)	14 (54%)
Total systems reporting	[N=6]	[N=15]	[N=26]

Table 9

Type of corporate relationships with nursing in member hospitals.

Type of Relationship	Multihospital System: Centralized NCL	Decentralized NCL	Decentralized NNCL
Corporate headquarters	4	14	4
Regional office	1	1	4
Other:			
Hospital administrator	0	0	1
Nursing consultant	0	0	1
Coordinating CEO	0	0	1
Informal network	0	0	1
Management company arm	0	1	0
Direct request only	1	0	0
No answer	0	0	14

Of the total respondents, 60 percent of centralized systems and 80 percent of decentralized systems with an NCL indicated consistent nursing input into corporate policy, compared with 23 percent of decentralized systems with no NCL (as shown in Table 10a).

In centralized systems, member hospital nurses provided input through a corporate nursing staff. In decentralized systems, input is provided through a nursing advisory committee or ad hoc committee of directors of nursing.

Table 10a

Respondents' perceptions about nursing input into corporate policy.

	Multihospital System					
	N=5 Centralized NCL		N=15 Decentralized NCL		N=26 NNCL	
	#	%	#	%	#	%
Consistently	3	60	12	80	6	23
Sometimes	1	20	1	7	10	38
Rarely	1	20	2	13	5	19
Never	0	0	0	0	2	8
No answer	0	0	0	0	3	12

Format for Nursing Input into Corporate Policy Decisions

The majority of respondents that reported presence of a format for nursing input into corporate policy decisions indicated that this input was provided by management teams, followed in order of frequency by committee participation and surveys. All formats reported are shown in Table 10b.

The extent of nursing input indicated by respondents varied, with 45 percent giving no answer to whether input was limited to nursing or general to the corporation. An overview of responses is shown in Table 10c.

Table 10b

Format for nursing input into corporate policy decisions by type of organization.

	Multihospital System							
			Decentralized					
	N=5 Centralized NCL		N=15 NCL		N=26 NNCL		N=47 Total	
Format	#	%	#	%	#	%	#	%
Management Team	3	60	14	93	7	27	24	51
Committee Participation	1	20	10	67	12	46	23	50
Survey	1	20	6	40	3	12	10	21
Hospital Administration	–	–	1	7	3	12	4	9
Incidental	1	20	–	–	–	–	1	2
Informal	–	–	–	–	1	4	1	2
Nursing Council	–	–	1	7	–	–	1	2
Review at Division Level	–	–	–	–	1	4	1	2
Report to Governing Board	–	–	1	7	–	–	1	2

Table 10c

Extent of nursing input to the corporation by type of organization.

	Multihospital System									
	Centralized				Decentralized					
	N=5 NCL		N=1 NNCL		N=15 NCL		N=26 NNCL		N=47 Total	
Extent of Input	#	%	#	%	#	%	#	%	#	%
General to the Corporation	3	60	0	0	10	67	5	19	19	40
Limited to Nursing	1	20	1	100	3	20	13	50	18	38
Both	1	20	0	–	2	13	2	8	6	11
No Answer	0	–	0	–	0	0	6	23	6	11

Nature of Relationship between Corporate Headquarters and Nursing in Member Hospitals

The nature of the relationship between corporate headquarters and nursing in member hospitals was indicated by 31 respondents. Consultation was the most frequently mentioned response, followed by on request only in systems with no NCL and oversight in systems with an NCL. The total responses are shown in Table 11.

Table 11

Nature of relationship of corporation to member hospitals by category of organization and NCL.

	Multihospital System									
	Centralized				Decentralized					
	NCL		NNCL		NCL		NNCL		Total	
	#	%	#	%	#	%	#	%	#	%
Direct Management	2	40	0	0	1	7	0	0	3	5
Oversight	–	–	0	0	8	53	3	12	11	23
Consultation	5	100	0	0	14	93	6	23	25	53
On Request Only	3	60	1	100	2	13	11	42	11	34
Other:										
Direction From Central Office	0	0	–	–	–	–	–	–	–	–
Routine Visits	1	20	–	–	–	–	–	–	1	2
None	1	20	–	–	2	13	14	54	16	34

Nursing Department Data Routinely Received by Corporate Office from Member Hospital

Another aspect of the relationship between the corporate office and nursing in member hospitals queried was the type of nursing data routinely received by the corporate office from member hospitals. Table 12 provides the categories of information received.

Table 12

Data routinely received from member hospitals by corporate office.

	Multihospital System							
	Centralized		Decentralized				N=47	
	NCL		NCL		NNCL		Total	
Format	#	%	#	%	#	%	#	%
Nursing Hours Per Patient Day	5	100	12	87	12	46	30	64
Nursing Department Budget	5	100	10	67	14	54	29	62
Nurse-Patient Ratio	4	80	10	67	10	38	24	51
Staff Nurse Turnover Rate	2	40	9	60	8	31	19	40
Staff Nurse Vacancy Rate	3	60	8	53	8	31	19	40
Nursing Care Audit	3	60	8	53	8	31	13	28
Registry Use	1	20	1	6	1	4	3	6
Continuing Education Program Goals and Objectives	–	–	1	6	–	–	–	–
Incident Reports	–	–	2	13	–	–	–	–
Policy Changes	–	–	1	6	–	–	–	–
Quality Assurance Projects	–	–	1	6	–	–	–	–

Standardization

The amount of standardization reported was minimal, as shown in Table 13. Of respondents reporting standardized policies, procedures or forms, decentralized systems with an NCL had the greatest number. Overall, the extent of standardization reported was variable.

Relationship to Nursing Schools

In the total sample, 28 systems had hospitals that provided clinical experience for licensed practical nurse students, 24 for associate degree nurse students, 29 for baccalaureate degree nurse students and 10 for higher degree nurse students. One system reported that seven hospitals in the system operated nine diploma programs and one had two diploma programs at the corporate level. Licensed practical nurse programs were operated by one multisystem hospital and two corporations.

Agreements or clinical affiliations with schools of nursing were reported for both corporate and hospital levels, as shown in Table 14. Standard agreements were indicated for clinical experience, graduate RN education and research and development.

Financial support provided by multihospital systems at either the corporate or hospital level was in the form of program subsidy, faculty positions or student aid through tuition reimbursement, scholarships or loans. More than half of the respondents indicated that they provided some form of support to nursing schools. Scholarships, student loans, and student tuition were the most frequently provided form of support. All forms of support were provided more frequently by hospitals with the systems than by the corporation (see Table 15).

Table 13

Standardized policies, procedures and forms.

	Multihospital System							
			Decentralized					
Standardized Policies, Procedures, or Forms	**N=5 Centralized NCL**		**N=15 NCL**		**N=26 NNCL**		**N=47 Total**	
	#	%	#	%	#	%	#	%
Department Classification System	3	60	5	33	3	12	11	23
Nursing Department Policies	0	0	6	40	0	0	6	13
Standards of Care	0	0	4	27	0	0	4	9
Nursing Care Plan Forms	0	0	3	20	0	0	3	6
Continuing Education	1	20	1	7	0	0	2	4
Chart Forms	1	20	0	0	1	4	2	4
Nursing Quality Goals	0	0	1	7	0	0	1	2
Guidelines for Individualization	0	0	0	0	1	4	1	2
Orientation for Nurse Administrator	0	0	1	7	0	0	1	2
Quality Assurance	0	0	1	7	0	0	1	2

Table 14

Standard agreements with schools of nursing by type of organizations.

	Multihospital System									
	Centralized				Decentralized					
	N=5 NCL		**N=1 NNCL**		**N=15 NCL**		**N=26 NNCL**		**N=47 Total**	
Standard Agreement	#	%	#	%	#	%	#	%	#	%
Clinical Experience										
■ Hospital	3	60	0	0	9	60	15	57	27	57
■ Corporation	0	0	1	100	5	33	5	19	11	23
Graduate Education										
■ Hospital	2	40	0	0	7	47	7	30	16	34
■ Corporation	0	0	1	100	3	20	2	8	6	13
Research & Development										
■ Hospital	2	40	0	0	5	33	7	30	14	30
■ Corporation	0	0	1	100	6	40	1	6	8	17

Table 15

Financial support to nursing schools or students by type of organization and support.

	Multihospital System									
	Centralized				Decentralized					
	N=5 NCL		N=1 NNCL		N=15 NCL		N=26 NNCL		N=47 Total	
Support To Schools/Students	#	%	#	%	#	%	#	%	#	%
Provide Support										
▪ Yes	3	60	1	100	10	67	12	80	26	55
▪ No	2	40	0	0	4	27	8	31	14	30
Type of Support to Schools										
▪ Program Subsidy										
hosp. level	1	10	0	0	6	40	10	38	17	36
corp. level	0	0	1	100	5	33	1	4	7	15
▪ Faculty Positions										
hosp. level	1	–	1	100	4	27	7	27	13	28
corp. level	0	0	0	–	1	7	1	4	2	4
Type of Support to Students										
▪ Tuition										
hosp. level	3	60	0	0	8	53	7	27	18	38
corp. level	0	0	0	0	7	47	4	15	11	23
▪ Scholarships										
hosp. level	2	40	0	0	8	53	9	35	19	40
corp. level	0	0	1	100	5	33	3	12	9	19
▪ Loans										
hosp. level	2	40	0	0	7	47	9	35	18	38
corp. level	0	0	1	100	2	12	0	0	3	6

Interpretation and Recommendations

The data reported are limited to 16 percent of the multihospital systems listed in the *Directory of Multihospital Systems,* 1982. This 16 percent represented 44 percent of the hospitals and 36 percent of the beds listed for all systems in the directory, indicating the wide range in size of multihospital systems. Postcards identifying a person or title at the corporate level responsible for nursing were returned from 178 systems. Surveys were sent to all 178 systems and 47 were returned, a 26 percent response rate. An unrecorded number of additional systems indicated that the survey did not apply to their system. It is not known whether the remaining multihospital systems considered the survey non-applicable or whether those systems simply did not respond to the survey.

Most of the respondents with an NCL initiated this position within six years prior to the survey, indicating the relative newness of corporate nursing. Two multihospital systems that responded have employed an NCL since the survey was completed. This position may evolve as multihospitals grow. That only 43 percent of the respondents employed an NCL may indicate that this position is evolving as multihospital systems evolve.

The respondents represent a cross-section of multihospital systems by type of organizational control, size and geographic distribution. Data from the survey thus provide insight into the early development of corporate nursing and into the relationship between nursing in member hospitals and corporate headquarters. The data indicate that organizational control and size do not seem to be major factors influencing the way nursing in member hospitals relates to the corporate office.

Responses from this survey indicate that nursing departments in member hospitals were most influenced by corporate functions related to management education and consultation, personnel recruitment, compensation, benefits, nursing department policy, quality assurance and risk management. These functions appear to be more frequently provided by centralized and decentralized multihospital systems with an NCL. The survey did not differentiate between functions provided by contract-managed or owned, leased or sponsored hospitals. Only four respondents had only contract-managed hospitals.

The high number of corporate nursing functions (48 percent) related to nursing department policy is interesting when related to the relatively low number (13 percent) of standardized nursing department policies reported. The definition of nursing department policies needs to be further explored to explain the corporate nursing role in relation to member hospitals. These data imply that the NCL deals with member hospitals on a highly individualized basis.

Corporate functions appear to be supportive and developmental for nursing departments in member hospitals. Management education and consultation were the most frequently reported functions, while presence of standardized policies, procedures or forms reported was negligible. The data also indicate an oversight role of corporations. Quality assurance and risk management were frequently mentioned functions. Data routinely received by corporate offices from member hospitals regarding nursing were also related to oversight, budgetary and personnel data, nurse-patient ratio or nursing hours per patient day. The concern for quality patient care was indicated by the function "quality assurance" and data about nursing care audits routinely received by corporate offices.

Committee participation appeared to be strong in the relationship between corporate offices and member hospitals. The data indicate that the majority of respondents felt that nursing input into corporation policies was consistent or sometimes consistent. Committees, particularly committees of directors of nursing from member hospitals, were noted by respondents to be related to their opportunity for nursing input. There appeared to be a clearer perception of the relationships between the corporation and nursing in member hospitals in centralized and decentralized systems with an NCL. (Only one of the respondents from centralized systems did not have an NCL.) Fewer responses to questions concerning the nature of the relationship and fewer formats for input into corporate policy were reported by respondents from decentralized systems with no NCL.

It was interesting to note that more than 50 percent of the respondents with an NCL indicated that nursing input was general to the corporation rather than limited to nursing. This finding can be interpreted to mean that nursing in systems with an NCL perceives a greater identity with the corporation than in those without an NCL, or that the NCL is more involved in corporate policy, or both. Decentralized systems and those with an NCL also appear to be more involved with nursing education, research and development than in those with no NCL, even though those areas were frequently reported to be member hospital arrangements rather than corporate arrangements.

SUMMARY

Results of this survey indicate trends in nursing's relationship to multihospital systems.

These data, for example, suggest that corporations relate to nursing departments in member hospitals in matters of governance, administration and management. There is no evidence that multihospital systems represented in this sample have directly affected the clinical practice of nursing in hospitals. In this perspective, corporations appear to have separated governance and administrative policy issues from the issues of nursing as a clinical practice discipline. This separation may be useful to nurse administrators in hospitals who are involved in the transition of nursing practice from the task-structured mode to the current clinical practice mode.

Nurse administrators in hospitals and corporate offices interface between the clinical practice of nursing and governance and administration of hospitals. Their functions are changing as they become more involved in the policy formulation and institutional decision making inherent in their role as an executive management team member. The results of this survey thus begin to clarify the functions of nurse administrators. The functions identified have implications for evaluation and development of graduate nursing curricula needed to educate nurse administrators.

Results of this survey are not definitive but point the way for further study. Questions most cogent to the nurse administrator's role and also to the relationship between corporate nursing and member hospital nursing departments are: 1) How does corporate nursing relate to member hospital nursing department policy? and 2) What administrative and management tools can be used or developed to ensure efficient and cost-effective quality nursing care in member hospitals?

This survey was limited to corporate-level responses. Further study of the relationship between member hospitals and corporations must involve nurses and others from both settings to obtain a more realistic perspective. For example, the results of this survey indicate that about 50 percent of the respondents thought nursing sometimes or consistently had input to corporate policy. This perception needs to be tested in member hospitals. Multihospital systems that have positive relationships and are also efficient could then be identified to examine organizational and administrative features that promote effective relationships and quality, cost-effective nursing care.

This survey is an early effort to examine and clarify the roles and functions of nurses in corporate level positions and to describe the relationship between corporations and nursing departments in member hospitals. As indicated by the survey results, there is diversity in philosophy, organization and administration in multihospital systems. The literature about multihospital systems indicates that they will continue to be developed. At best, this survey establishes a baseline for ongoing study. The variety of multihospital systems and the environments of change will make further study even more important in the effort to explain how organizations and people adapt to new circumstances and to burgeoning external and internal influences.

Appendix

2

NATIONAL NURSING ORGANIZATIONS

Membership of nurses in professional organizations and the varied national nursing organizations in the United States was discussed in responses to the *Initial Report and Preliminary Recommendations.* To clarify the phrase "national nursing organizations," the commission conducted a survey of national nursing organizations in November/December 1982. Thirty-two nursing organizations provided information about membership criteria, services, official publications, membership and other pertinent information summarized in this section.

The national nursing organizations listed alphabetically in this section have varied purposes and membership criteria. Types of membership were: institutional (3); institutional plus associates (1); registered nurses (13); registered nurses with associate membership for licensed practical nurses (2); registered nurses with open associate membership (5); licensed nurses including registered nurses and licensed practical nurses (2); open membership (5); and student nurses (1).

Official Name	American Academy of Nursing
Headquarters Address	2420 Pershing Road Kansas City, MO 64108
Telephone Number	816/474-5720
Director or Administrator	Vernice Ferguson President (until 9-27-83) Carolyn A. Williams President (from 9-27-83 to 9-27-85)
Criteria for Membership	RNs must be recommended by an AAN fellow, meet membership criteria and be elected by the AAN fellows.
Major Purposes	• Advancing new concepts in nursing and health care. • Exploring issues in health as they affect the development of the nursing profession.

	• Identifying and proposing resolutions to issues and problems.
Major Services Provided	• Annual scientific session • Quarterly newsletter • Publications • Symposias
Official Publications	• Academy Newsletter (quarterly)
Total Number of Members	• 451 (+18 honorary fellows)
Additional Information	The American Academy of Nursing is governed by a governing council composed of four officers and six fellows.

Official Name	American Association of Colleges of Nursing
Headquarters Address	11 Dupont Circle, Suite 430 Washington, DC 20036
Telephone Number	202/332-1917
Director or Administrator	Marion I. Murphy, R.N., Ph.D. Executive Director
Criteria for Membership	Institutions offering baccalaureate and higher degree programs in nursing. Membership is institutional, with dean as official representative.
Major Purposes	• To advance quality of baccalaureate and higher degree programs. • To promote research in nursing. • To develop academic leaders.
Major Services Provided	• Salary surveys annually for faculty, deans and other administrators in schools of nursing • Current update on nursing and health legislation • Forums for deans via semi-annual membership meetings • Monograph series
Official Publications	• AACN Newsletter (monthly) • Publication Series (four times per year) • Annual Report (yearly) • Institutional Data System (salary reports; other special reports for AACN member schools)
Total Number of Members	336
Additional Information	AACN has operated a federally funded project for four years entitled "Continuing Education for Academic Administrators." The project also operates a subscription series known as *Briefly Noted,* which digests pertinent books or articles for nursing administrators in education or practice.

Official Name	American Association of Critical-Care Nurses (AACN)
Headquarters Address	One Civic Plaza Newport Beach, CA 92660
Telephone Number	714/644-9310
Director or Administrator	Dr. Edward A. Shaw Executive Director

Criteria for Membership	• Registered professional nurses hold active status • Licensed Vocational Nurses, Licensed Practical Nurses and students in Registered Nurse, Licensed Vocational Nurse or Licensed Practical Nurse programs hold associate status
Major Purposes	• To promote the health and welfare of mankind by advancing the science and art of critical care nursing. • To provide education to critical care nurses, promote professionalism and accountability among critical care nurses, facilitate effective communication within the profession and with the public and encourage scientific investigation in critical care.
Major Services Provided	• Educational opportunities (formal programs, multi-media programs, publication of textbooks and other learning aids, individual membership benefits such as group life insurance, disability income and professional liability insurance) • Certification through separate affiliate corporation (also open to non-member critical care nurses)
Official Publications	• *Focus on Critical Care* (six times per year) • *Heart & Lung: The Journal of Critical Care* (six times per year)
Total Number of Members	46,000 individual members
Additional Information	AACN is the world's largest specialty nursing organization. Approximately 200 local chapters are organized. AACN pursues active liaison relationships with many other specialty organizations, physician associations and government agencies.

Official Name	American Association of Nephrology Nurses & Technicians
Headquarters Address	North Woodbury Road, Box 56 Pitman, NJ 08071
Telephone Number	609/589-2187
Director or Administrator	Ron Brady Executive Director
Criteria for Membership	• Full Member: Registered Nurses, Licensed Practical/Vocational Nurses, Technician • Associate Member: Social Worker, Dietitian, Physician, Industry
Major Purposes	The American Association of Nephrology Nurses & Technicians has the obligation to set forth and update high standards of patient care, educate its practitioners, stimulate research, disseminate new ideas throughout the field, promote interdisciplinary communication and cooperation and address issues encompassing the practice of nephrology nursing and technology.

Major Services Provided	• Four regional meetings per year • One annual meeting • Standards of clinical practice • Position papers on role of the Registered Nurse, Licensed Practical Nurse and dialysis technician • Transplantation, self-dialysis, renal osteodystrophy and peritoneal dialysis monographs • Group insurance program
Official Publications	• *AANNT Newsletter* (bi-monthly) • *AANNT Journal* (bi-monthly)
Total Number of Members	3,683

Official Name	American Association of Neuroscience Nurses
Headquarters Address	625 North Michigan Avenue, Suite 1519 Chicago, IL 60611
Telephone Number	312/944-4280
Director or Administrator	Rita Shafer Executive Secretary
Criteria for Membership	Registered nurses licensed in United States or Canada
Major Purposes	To foster and promote interest, education and high standards of practice in the specialty.
Major Services Provided	• Annual meeting • Continuing education approval • Journal, insurance programs, regional chapters • Development of materials in areas such as research and standards of practice
Official Publications	• *Synapse* (bi-monthly) • *Journal of Neurosurgical Nursing* (bi-monthly)
Total Number of Members	1,600 individual members
Additional Information	• Developed and published two cores as resource material for the neurological/neurosurgical nurse: Clinical Core Curriculum (1977, revision due in 1983) and Core Curriculum for Neurosurgical Nursing in the Operating Room (1980). • Established a credible speakers' bureau of neuro nurse experts (available to regional chapters and other interested parties). • Member organization and active participant of the National Federation for Specialty Nursing Organizations and closely affiliated with ABNN, an organization that administers certification process for neurological/neurosurgical nurses.

Official Name	American Association of Nurse Anesthetists
Headquarters Address	216 Higgins Road Park Ridge, IL 60068
Telephone Number	312/692-7050
Director or Administrator	Nancy A. Fevold Executive Director
Criteria for Membership	Registered Nurses only

Major Purposes	Members are committed to the advancement of educational standards and practices which will advance the art and science of anesthesiology and thereby support and enhance quality patient care.
Major Services Provided	• Promote continual high-quality patient care. • Advance the science and art of anesthesiology. • Develop and promote educational standards in the field of nurse anesthesia. • Facilitate effective cooperation between nurse anesthetists, anesthesiologists and other members of the medical profession, the nursing profession, hospitals and agencies representing a community of interest in nurse anesthesia. • Publish scientific journals, bulletins and other publications pertinent to the objectives of the Association. • Maintain informational and statistical data for reference and assistance in matters pertaining to the profession or its practice. • Provide opportunities for continuing education in anesthesia. • Provide members with direction pertaining to governmental policy, legislation or judicial decisions of importance to anesthesia.
Official Publications	• *AANA News Bulletin* (monthly) • *AANA Journal* (bi-monthly) • *AANA Fact Book* • *Anesthesia: A Special Kind of Nursing* • List of Schools
Total Number of Members	18,620

Official Name	American Association of Occupational Health Nurses
Headquarters Address	3500 Piedmont Road, Suite 400 Atlanta, GA 30305
Telephone Number	404/262-1162
Director or Administrator	Matilda A. Babbitz Executive Director
Criteria for Membership	Registered Nurses only
Major Purposes	• To constitute the professional association of nurses engaged in the practice of occupational health nursing. • To promote and provide continuing education in occupational health nursing for members. • To maintain the honor and character of the nursing profession. • To improve community health by bettering nursing service to workers. • To develop and promote standards for occupational health nurses and occupational health nursing services.

- To stimulate interest in and provide a forum for the discussion of problems in the field of occupational health nursing.
- To stimulate occupational health nurse participation in all nursing activities—local, state and national.
- To do within the limits of the law all things necessary, proper, incidental, suitable, useful and conducive to the complete accomplishment of the foregoing purposes.

Services Provided	• Educational opportunities • Legislative information • Conferences • Journal
Official Publications	• *AAOHN Newsletter* (monthly) • *Occupational Health Nursing* (monthly)
Total Number of Members	11,600+

Official Name	American Colleges of Nurse-Midwives
Headquarters Address	1522 K Street, N.W. Washington, DC 20005
Telephone Number	202/347-5445
Director or Administrator	Florence McGregor McDaniel Administrative Director
Criteria for Membership	Certified nurse-midwives

Major Purposes

- To study, develop and evaluate standards for nurse-midwifery care of women and infants.
- To study, develop and evaluate standards for nurse-midwifery education.
- To support and assist in the development of nurse-midwifery services and educational programs, in association with allied professional groups.
- To evaluate and approve nurse-midwifery services and educational programs.
- To determine the eligibility of individuals to practice as certified nurse-midwives and to assume responsibility for national nurse-midwifery certification.
- To facilitate and coordinate the efforts of nurse-midwives who in the public interest provide quality services to individuals and childbearing families.
- To establish channels for communication and cooperation with other professional and non-professional groups who in the public interest share the objectives of ensuring sufficient quality services to individuals and childbearing families.
- To establish channels for interpretation of nurse-midwifery to allied professional and non-professional groups on a regional, national and international basis.

	• To promote research and the development of literature in the field of nurse-midwifery.
Major Services Provided	• Publications • Annual convention • Continuing education • Lobbying activities • Liability insurance
Official Publications	• *Quickening* (bi-monthly) • *Journal of Nurse-Midwifery* (bi-monthly)
Total Number of Members	2,600

Official Name	American Nurses' Association
Headquarters Address	2420 Pershing Road Kansas City, MO 64108
Telephone Number	816/474-5720
Director or Administrator	Judith A. Ryan Executive Director
Criteria for Membership	Constituent state nurses' associations (SNAs) who provide that each member has either: • been granted a license to practice as a registered nurse in at least one state, territory or possession of the United States and does not have a license under suspension or revocation in any state; or • completed a nursing education program qualifying the individual to take the state-recognized examination for registered nurse licensure as a first-time writer.
Major Purposes	• To work for the improvement of health standards and the availability of health care services for all people. • To foster high standards of nursing. • To stimulate and promote the professional development of nurses and advance their economic and general welfare. • (The purposes shall be unrestricted by consideration of nationality, race, creed, lifestyle, color, sex or age).
Major Services Provided	• Establish standards of nursing practice, nursing education and nursing services. • Establish a code of ethical conduct for nurses. • Ensure a system of credentialing in nursing. • Initiate and influence legislation, governmental programs, national health policy and international health policy. • Support systematic study, evaluation and research in nursing. • Serve as a central agency for the collection, analysis and dissemination of information relevant to nursing. • Promote and protect the economic and general welfare of nurses. • Provide leadership in national and international nursing.

	• Provide for the professional development of nurses. • Conduct an affirmative action program. • Ensure a collective bargaining program for nurses. • Provide services to constituent state nurses' associations. • Maintain communication with members through official publications. • Assume an active role as consumer advocate. • Represent and speak for the nursing profession with allied health groups, national and international organizations, governmental bodies and the public.
Official Publications	• *The American Nurse* (10 times per year) • *American Journal of Nursing* (monthly)
Total Number of Members	163,761 SNA/ANA

Official Name	American Society for Nursing Service Administrators
Headquarters Address	840 North Lake Shore Drive Chicago, IL 60611
Telephone Number	312/280-6410
Director or Administrator	Janine A. Swent Director
Criteria for Membership	• Registered nurses currently in management positions (top level) in health care institutions • Affiliates
Major Purposes	To advance the development of effective administration in nursing service in health care institutions and provide a platform for NSAs to speak on nursing and health issues.
Major Services Provided	• Medium for interchange of ideas • Publications and materials relative to nursing service administration • Educational programs • Recognition program
Official Publications	• *Nursing Service Administration* (6 times per year)
Total Number of Members	• 3,200 individual members • 45 affiliated chapters

Official Name	American Society of Ophthalmic Registered Nurses, Inc.
Headquarters Address	c/o American Academy of Ophthalmology 1833 Fillmore Street, P.O. Box 3030 San Francisco, CA 94120
Telephone Number	415/921-4700
Director or Administrator	Susan Brown Administrator
Criteria for Membership	Registered Nurses only
Major Purposes	• Education of ophthalmic Registered Nurses in field to existing knowledge.

	• Continuing education.
Major Services Provided	• Annual meeting (3 days) • Newsletter
Official Publications	*Insight* (6 times per year)
Total Number of Members	704
Additional Information	Formed in 1976 from a core of 24 members.

Official Name	American Society of Post Anesthesia Nurses
Headquarters Address	P.O. Box 11083 2405 Westwood Avenue, Suite 200 Richmond, VA 23230
Telephone Number	804/359-3557
Director or Administrator	John A. Hinckley Executive Secretary
Criteria for Membership	Nurses holding a recognized state license
Major Purposes	To promote education.
Major Services Provided	• General information on recovery room activities • Insurance
Official Publications	*Breathline* (4 times per year)
Total Number of Members	3,000
Additional Information	Developing a certification program and standards of care. Both should be completed in 1983.

Official Name	American Urological Association, Allied
Headquarters Address	6845 Lake Shore Drive P.O. Box 9397 Raytown, MO 64133
Telephone Number	816/358-3317
Director or Administrator	Bruce Hagen President Ardeth S. Hale, C.U.R.N. Executive Secretary
Criteria for Membership	RNs, LPNs, Technicians, PAs, MDs
Major Purposes	• To engender a high quality of urological education for urological allied health professionals. • To unite these professionals for the purpose of maintaining an association dedicated to the promotion of the highest professional standards for the better and safer care of the urologic patient. • To study, discuss and exchange information in the field of urology. • To hold meetings at intervals for the purpose of the AUAA.
Major Services Provided	• Annual assembly • Discounted registration fees for local, regional or national seminars • Resource for urologic information • Official publications provided to members at no charge

Official Publications	• *Uro-Gram* (quarterly) • Section Newsletters (quarterly) • *The AUAA Journal* (quarterly) • *Standards of Urologic Nursing Practice* (published in conjunction with the ANA in 1977)
Total Number of Members	1,246 (RN, 665; LPN, 112; LVN, 11; PA, 15; Tech., 32; UT, 67; ET, 2; MD, 8; Indust. Rep., 26; NonCat., 101; CURN, 138; CULPN, 10; CULVN, 1; CUPA, 10; CUT, 48)
Additional Information	• Certifying board since 1972. • Re-certification for all who have been certified for five years or longer. • 32 chapters. • Charter member of the National Federation of Specialty Nursing Organizations. • Recognized by the American Urological Association as the official provider of continuing education for urological allied health professionals.

Official Name	Assembly of Hospital Schools of Nursing
Headquarters Address	840 North Lake Shore Drive Chicago, Illinois 60611
Telephone Number	312/280-6633
Director or Administrator	Carol A. Boston, R.N. Director
Criteria for Membership	• Two members per institution • C.E.O. of affiliating hospital • Director of school • Institution must be a member of the American Hospital Association
Major Purposes	• To maintain the viability of hospital schools of nursing as providers of professional nursing education. • To assist schools in the development of articulation models. • To provide representation, advocacy and programmatic services to membership.
Official Publications	• *Hospital Schools of Nursing* (6 times per year) • *State Group Informational Update* (3 times per year)
Total Number of Members	• Individual members: 486 • Institutional members: 243

Official Name	Association for Practitioners in Infection Control
Headquarters Address	23341 North Milwaukee Avenue Half Day, IL 60069
Telephone Number	312/634-1403
Director or Administrator	Edward J. Stygar, Jr. Executive Director
Criteria for Membership	Multidisciplinary. Registered Nurses, physicians, microbiologists, epidemiologists, medical technicians

Major Purposes	To improve patient care by serving the needs and aims common to all disciplines who are united in infection control.
Major Services Provided	• Subscription to journal • Annual educational conference • Local programs
Official Publications	*American Journal of Infection Control* (bi-monthly)
Total Number of Members	Approximately 6,000

Official Name	Association of Diploma Schools of Professional Nursing
Headquarters Address	Center for Health Affairs 760 Alexander Road Princeton, NJ 08540
Telephone Number	609/452-9280
Director or Administrator	Eileen J. Alessandro Executive Director
Criteria for Membership	• Diploma schools, their faculty and registered nurses • Associate membership for other nursing programs with strong hospital affiliations
Major Services Provided	• Monitoring nursing organizations and boards. • Newsletter publication • Continuing education • Lobbying and legislative reviews • Making public position statements on nursing issues. • Recruitment of students
Official Publications	• *Nursing First* (2-4 times per year) • *We're Nurses First* (recruitment catalog of all diploma schools in the state) • *We're Nurses First* (poster for student recruitment)
Total Number of Members	• 18 schools • 250 individual members (fluctuates) • New individual membership drive to be completed in July 1983 for Registered Nurses outside the hospital schools.

Official Name	The Association of Operating Room Nurses, Inc.
Headquarters Address	10170 East Mississippi Avenue Denver, CO 80231
Telephone Number	303/755-6300
Director or Administrator	Clifford H. Jordan Executive Director
Criteria for Membership	Registered Nurses only
Major Purposes	• To unite registered professional operating room nurses for the purpose of maintaining an Association dedicated to promoting highest professional standards of operating room nursing for the optimum care of the patient before, during and after surgery.

	• To study, discuss and exchange information in the field of operating room nursing. • To hold meetings at intervals for the purpose of this Association. • To cooperate lawfully with other professional associations, hospitals, universities, industries, technical societies, research organizations and governmental agencies in matters affecting the foregoing purpose of the Association. • To provide for the continuing education of nurses whose practice centers in the nation's operating suites. • To conduct national educational seminars. • To hold an annual Congress. • Education.
Official Publications	• *AORN Newsletter* (monthly) • *INFORM* (quarterly) • *AORN Journal* (13 issues annually)
Total Number of Members	28,809 individual members

Official Name	Association of Rehabilitation Nurses
Headquarters Address	2506 Gross Point Road Evanston, IL 60201
Telephone Number	312/475-7530
Director or Administrator	Dagny N. Engle Executive Director
Criteria for Membership	• Voting membership: Registered Nurses only • Non-voting membership: any individual interested in rehabilitation nursing
Major Purposes	To advance the quality of rehabilitation nursing service throughout the community by offering educational opportunities and facilitating the exchange of ideas in rehabilitation programs.
Major Services Provided	• National educational conference • Regional seminars • Chapter workshops • Publications • Subscription to *Rehabilitation Nursing* journal • Professional liability insurance • Investigation of certification of rehabilitation nurses
Official Publications	• *Rehabilitation Nursing* (bi-monthly) • *Standards of Rehabilitation Nursing Practice* • *Rehabilitation Nursing & Related Readings: A Bibliography* • *Rehabilitation Nursing: Concepts & Practice—A Core Curriculum*
Total Number of Members	2,200 individual members
Additional Information	Comprised of professional rehabilitation nurses from a variety of practice settings, including general hospitals, rehabilitation and long-term care facilities, insurance companies, educational institu-

tions and private consulting companies. Clinical practice interests encompass the broad spectrum of rehabilitation nursing.

Official Name	Drug and Alcohol Nursing Association, Inc.
Headquarters Address	P.O. Box 371 College Park, MD 20740
Telephone Number	202/541-7194
Director or Administrator	Frances S. Lewis President
Criteria for Membership	• Active members: Registered Nurses and Licensed Practical Nurses • Associate (non-voting) members: Interested parties in the health care field
Major Purposes	• To promote and maintain the involvement of the nursing profession in the addictions field. • To uphold the highest standards of nursing practice and nursing education. • To provide forums for discussion of issues in the drug and alcohol field. • To represent drug and alcohol nursing to allied professional groups, governmental bodies and the public.
Major Services Provided	• Annual meeting and conference • Education • Newsletter • Communication • Work with allied groups • Promotion of nurse role
Official Publications	*DANA Newsletter* (quarterly)
Total Number of Members	125 individual members
Additional Information	Nursing specialty organization established as an independent body to address the needs and concerns of nurses working in the drug and alcohol fields and to express these concerns to allied groups.

Official Name	Emergency Department Nurses Association
Headquarters Address	666 North Lake Shore Drive, Suite 1131 Chicago, IL 60611
Telephone Number	312/649-0297
Director or Administrator	Torry Mark Sansone Executive Director
Criteria for Membership	• Registered Nurses • Licensed Practical Nurses, EMTs, other health care professionals in the emergency setting
Major Purposes	• To develop and promote emergency health care public education programs. • To serve as patient advocate for the consumer. • To monitor emergency care quality assurance. • To interface with all areas involved with the emergency setting.

Major Services Provided	• Certified emergency nurse examination • Annual scientific assembly • Nursing practice issues • Continuing education programs • CECH maintenance • Accreditation
Official Publications	• *ET CETERA* (quarterly) • *Journal of Emergency Nursing* (bi-monthly) • *The Core Curriculum* (1980)
Total Number of Members	Approximately 11,000

Official Name	Federation of Independent Nursing Organizations
Headquarters Address	760 Alexander Road Princeton, NJ 08540
Telephone Number	609/452-9280
Director or Administrator	Christine Barney President
Criteria for Membership	Nurses interested in maintaining emphasis on clinical preparation
Major Purposes	• Share and disseminate information on nursing issues. • Promote involvement of nurses in issues. • Promote educational mobility opportunities for all nurses. • Support educational programs for nursing that emphasize clinical preparation and academic excellence.
Major Services Provided	• Meetings • Newsletters • Educational forums
Official Publications	Untitled (as needed)
Total Number of Members	26 (fluctuates from year to year)
Additional Information	Provides a national forum for small independent nursing organizations and groups to have a national voice and recognition through a national organization for support.

Official Name	International Association for Enterostomal Therapy
Headquarters Address	505 North Tustin Avenue, Suite 282 Santa Ana, CA 92705
Telephone Number	714/972-1720
Director or Administrator	Fred Droz Executive Director
Criteria for Membership	Several categories for membership
Major Purposes	The promotion of education to patients, nurses, physicians and other allied health professionals in the biopsychosocial and sexual rehabilitation of persons with abdominal stomas, fistulae, draining wounds, pressure sores and incontinence.

Major Services	• Provide and approve quality continuing education for nurses and other professionals in order to facilitate an ever-improving enterostomal therapy practice. • Certification program
Official Publications	• *Journal of Enterostomal Therapy* (bi-monthly) • *Enterostomal Therapy: A Nursing Specialty* (brochure) • *Accredited Professional Educational Programs* (brochure) • *Board Certification for Enterostomal Therapy* (brochure)
Total Number of Members	1,600

Official Name	National Association of Orthopaedic Nurses
Headquarters Address	North Woodbury Road P.O. Box 56 Pitman, NJ 08071
Telephone Number	609/582-0111
Director or Administrator	Mary Faut Rodts President
Criteria for Membership	• Registered Nurses • Licensed Practical Nurses • Licensed Vocation Nurses
Major Purposes	• To promote, in cooperation with all members of the health team, the highest standards of nursing practice. • To educate its practitioners. • To promote research.
Major Services Provided	• Local, district and national meetings • Publications
Official Publications	• *Newsletter of the National Association of Orthopaedic Nurses* (bi-monthly) • *Orthopaedic Nursing* (bi-monthly) • Monographs on topics chosen by the membership
Total Number of Members	3,479

Official Name	National Association of Pediatric Nurse Associates and Practitioners
Headquarters Address	North Woodbury Road P.O. Box 56 Pitman, NJ 08071
Telephone Number	609/589-5077
Director or Administrator	Mavis McGuire Executive Director
Criteria for Membership	• Pediatric nurse practitioners and associates certified by the National Board of Pediatric Nurse Practitioners and Associates • Registered Nurses who have completed a course which adheres to guidelines jointly developed by

	the ANA and AAP and subsequently endorsed by NAPNAP • Registered Nurses who are practicing as pediatric nurse practitioners or Associates and were trained prior to the established guidelines • Registered Nurses who are prepared as family nurse practitioners or school nurse practitioners • Registered Nurse faculty members who prepare the PNP/PNA, the family nurse practitioner and the school nurse practitioner
Major Purposes	Delivery of the highest quality health care to children.
Major Services Provided	• Educational opportunities accessible to all members through national and regional conferences and joint participation at the AAP meetings. • Annual conference
Official Publications	• *The Practitioner* (bi-monthly) • *Pediatric Nursing* (bi-monthly) • *Review of the Literature: Nurse Practitioners 1965–1979*
Total Number of Members	2,500

Official Name	National Association of Nurse Recruiters
Headquarters Address	111 East Wacker Drive, #600 Chicago, IL 60601
Telephone Number	312/644-6610
Director or Administrator	Martha A. DeGraaf Executive Director
Criteria for Membership	Nurse Recruiters (Associate category also available for other supportive individuals.)
Major Purposes	To promote and exchange sound and ethical principles of professional nurse recruitment which may be employed by its members for their mutual betterment and professional advancement. In order to achieve this, the Association seeks to maintain appropriate but separate relationships with voluntary and government hospitals, leading community health care organizations, educational institutions, nursing societies and all advertising media.
Major Services Provided	• Membership directory • NANR Newsletter • Bi-monthly information portfolio • Annual recruitment survey • Supplier and service resource directory • Annual conference (July) • Spring workshop (April)
Official Publications	• *NANR News* (bi-monthly) • *NANR Resource Directory* (annual) • *NANR Membership Directory* (annual) • *NANR Recruitment Survey* (annual)
Total Number of Members	• 1,390 individual members • 10 institutional members

Official Name	National Association of School Nurses, Inc.
Headquarters Address	7706 John Hancock Lane Dayton, OH 45459
Telephone Number	513/434-0008
Director or Administrator	Peggy Rufner Executive Director
Criteria for Membership	• Active Member: Registered Nurses actively employed by boards of education • Associate: Registered Nurses not eligible for active membership, but who work in schools
Major Purposes	• To promote and advance the quality of school health services and health education throughout the nation. • To operate as an educational organization.
Major Services Provided	• Continuing education program • Newsletter • Model guidelines for school nursing service • School nurse journal • Resolutions and position statements • Representation in the promotion of school health services by qualified nurses
Official Publications	• *NAS Newsletter* (4 times per year) • *School Nurse* (4 times per year) • *Guidelines for a Model School Nurse Services Program*
Total Number of Members	• Individual Members: 2,200 • Affiliated Groups: 34
Additional Information	• Provides leadership in the promotion of health services for all school children. • Speaks for the interests of school nurses to the nursing and health community and to the public. • Monitors legislation and keeps members informed of federal legislation pertaining to school health services. • Testifies regarding health legislation pertinent to school nursing and school health. • Promotes the specialty of school nursing. • Encourages research in school nursing. • Collaborates with other organizations in the promotion of school health issues.

Official Name	National Council of State Boards of Nursing
Headquarters Address	303 East Ohio Street, Suite 2010 Chicago, IL 60611
Telephone Number	312/329-1282
Director or Administrator	Eileen McQuaid Dvorak, Ph.D., R.N. Executive Director
Criteria for Membership	The Council consists of 59 member state boards that represent the public. Each member board has one delegate vote for each type of licensing examination it uses; registered nurse and licensed practical nurse licensing examination.

Major Purposes	• Provide a mechanism for all state boards to work together to promote the public health, safety and welfare through State Board activities for nursing licensure.
Major Services Provided	• Provides National Council Licensure Examination (formerly called the State Board Test Pool Exam). State boards contract for use of the examination and also nominate nurse item writers for preparing the examination. • Serves as an information source for boards. • Provides data related to licensure and nurse practice acts. • Conducts research and educational programs.
Official Publications	• *Newsletter to Member Boards* • *Publication Issues* (information of interest for free distribution)
Total Number of Members	59 member boards

Official Name	National Intravenous Therapy Association, Inc.
Headquarters Address	92 Concord Avenue, Suite 4 Belmont, MA 02178
Telephone Number	617/938-8547
Director or Administrator	Mary Larkin Executive Director
Criteria for Membership	• Active Members: RNs (93%) • Associate Members: MDs, Licensed Practical Nurses, R.Ph. (6%) • Corporate Members: Medical Industry (1%)
Major Purposes	• To provide the benefits and protection of a qualified IV nurse. • To assure high quality of professional practice. • To promote research and education in IV nursing practices and related areas. • To disseminate knowledge by providing for interchange of information among members.
Major Services Provided	• Journal • Newsletter • Annual convention • Local Chapter: 47 • Bi-monthly meetings • Nursing standards: general IV and TPN • Insurance programs • Certification (investigating)
Official Publications	• *NITA Update* (bi-monthly) • *NITA*, the official journal of the National Intravenous Therapy Association (bi-monthly)
Total Number of Members	• Active: 2,778 • Associate: 209
Additional Information	• Specialized IV nursing teams within institutions decrease patient complications and are cost-effective.

- The National Intravenous Therapy Association is also involved with home care through home intravenous and TPN programs.

Official Name	National League for Nursing
Headquarters Address	10 Columbus Circle New York, NY 10019
Telephone Number	212/582-1022
Director or Administrator	Pamela Maraldo Executive Director
Criteria for Membership	Open membership
Major Purposes	Developing and improving the standards of quality nursing education, nursing services and health care delivery in the United States.
Major Services Provided	• Accreditation • Consultation • Continuing education • Testing • Research • Publications • Public affairs
Official Publications	• Memos issued by each of NLN's member agency Councils • *Nursing and Health Care* • Approximately 400 titles included in NLN publications catalog (manuals, guides, monographs, workshop papers, etc.) • 100+ new/revised editions per year
Total Number of Members	• Individual Members: 15,500 • Institutional Members: 1,800 • State and Constituent Leagues: 47
Additional Information	• NLN is officially recognized as the national accrediting agency for nursing education programs. • NLN is a coalition of nurses, educators, consumers, other heatlh care professionals and health care administrators.

Official Name	National Student Nurses' Association
Headquarters Address	10 Columbus Circle New York, NY 10019
Telephone Number	212/581-2211
Director or Administrator	Mary Ann Tuft Executive Director
Criteria for Membership	RN student nurses
Major Purposes	• To assume responsibility for contributing to nursing education in order to provide for the highest quality health care. • To provide programs representative of fundamental and current professional interest and concerns.

	• To aid in the development of the whole person and his/her professional role, and his/her responsibility for the health care of people of all walks of life.
Major Services Provided	• Career planning seminars • Scholarship/work commitment grants • Updated information regarding legislation, education, community health
Official Publications	• *NSNA News* (7 times per year) • Legislative alerts, community health (when the need arises) • *Imprint* (5 times per year) • Dean's list [for educators] (5 times per year)
Total Number of Members	30,000 individual members
Additional Information	Only nursing association geared to students of nursing.

Official Name	Nurse Consultants Association
Headquarters Address	8 Markham Court Hockessin, DE 19707
Telephone Number	302/239-6225
Director or Administrator	None yet
Criteria for Membership	Registered Nurses only
Major Purposes	Communication and education link for nurses working in the health care business world.
Major Services Provided	• Semi-annual meetings • Educational programs • Professional network • Resource listing
Official Publications	*NCA Newsletter* (quarterly)
Total Number of Members	125 individual members
Additional Information	• Nurses working in all phases of the health care market. • Considering more formal structure with an executive director.

Official Name	The Nurses Association of the American College of Obstetricians and Gynecologists
Headquarters Address	600 Maryland Avenue, S.W., Suite 200 East Washington, DC 20024
Telephone Number	202/638-0026
Director or Administrator	Sallye P. Brown Executive Director
Criteria for Membership	• Full Member: Registered Nurse, graduate of accredited school of nursing, currently employed or expressed interest in obstetric, gynecologic, neonatal nursing • Associate Member: Allied health care provider actively involved in obstetric, gynecologic, neonatal nursing

Major Purposes	• Promote the highest standards of obstetric, gynecologic, neonatal nursing practice, education and research. • Cooperate with all members of the health team. • Stimulate interest in obstetric, gynecologic and neonatal nursing.
Major Services Provided	• OGN Standards • Practice Resources (3-4 annually) • Continuing education in a variety of formats (i.e., live courses offered regionally, videotapes, home study modules, national meetings) • Role descriptions/curriculum guidelines for nurses in the field • Three types of health insurance (disability, liability, life) • Journal and newsletter monthly and bi-monthly • Legislative networking
Official Publications	• *NAACOG Newsletter* (monthly) • *Advisory Council News* (6 issues per year) • *Journal of Obstetric, Gynecologic, Neonatal Nursing* (6 times per year)
Total Number of Members	17,500

Official Name	Oncology Nursing Society
Headquarters Address	701 Washington Road Pittsburgh, PA 15228
Telephone Number	412/344-3899
Director or Administrator	Pearl Moore Executive Director
Criteria for Membership	Registered Nurses only
Major Purposes	• Promote the highest professional standards of oncology nursing. • Study, research and exchange information, experiences and ideas leading to improved oncology nursing. • Encourage nurses to specialize in the practice of oncology nursing.
Major Services Provided	• Quarterly issues of the *Oncology Nursing Forum* • Annual congress • Outcome standards for cancer nursing practice • Outcome standards for cancer nursing education • Eligibility for membership in local chapters of the ONS • Membership directory
Official Publications	*Oncology Nursing Forum* (quarterly)
Total Number of Members	4,600

Official Name	Sigma Theta Tau, Inc.
Headquarters Address	610 Barnhill Drive Indianapolis, IN 46223
Telephone Number	317/264-4689

Director or Administrator	Nell J. Watts Executive Officer
Criteria for Membership	Students in baccalaureate and graduate nursing programs where chapters exist who have demonstrated excellence in their nursing programs. Graduates of baccalaureate programs demonstrating excellence in leadership positions in nursing are also eligible for membership consideration.
Major Purposes	• Recognize superior achievement. • Recognize the development of leadership qualities. • Foster high professional standards. • Encourage creative work. • Strengthen commitment to the ideals and purposes of the profession.
Major Services Provided	• Research grants program • Sponsors national research conferences at ANA and NLN biennial conventions • Educational programs at national and chapter levels
Official Publications	• *Reflections* (quarterly) • *Image* (quarterly) • Research monographs (periodically)
Total Number of Members	• 51,000 active individuals • 162 chapters • American College of Honor Societies

Appendix

3

MODELS FOR EDUCATIONAL TRANSITION: CONVERSION TO DEGREE-GRANTING STATUS

by Sharon B. Buchbinder

INTRODUCTION

Transition of nursing education into the mainstream of higher education in the United States has occurred in response to societal and technologic factors that have increased the knowledge and skill needed for nursing practice. One concern in this movement of diploma nursing education to collegiate, degree-based education is maintaining and expanding current resources for nursing education. Converting these resources to a degree-granting program is one approach being used in the transition to collegiate-based nursing education. This study of conversion of diploma nursing education programs to degree-granting status was conducted to examine and identify features of program administration and change that directors of nursing schools thought were essential and/or beneficial for change.

For the purposes of this study, a conversion program was defined as a diploma nursing program that has converted or is converting its educational resources to a degree-based nursing program.

Criteria for inclusion in the study as a conversion program were as follows:

- graduates receive an associate degree (ADN) or baccalaureate degree (BSN) in nursing and are eligible for registered nurse licensure;
- the resources of the diploma program were used in the new degree-based program; and
- the transition was initiated or completed within the past 10 years.

Methodology

The National League for Nursing was contacted to obtain the names of schools of nursing that met these criteria. Additional names were obtained as the survey progressed. No attempt was made to locate all such programs; it is recognized that there

---

Sharon B. Buchbinder is staff specialist for the Division of Nursing, American Hospital Association.

may be other programs that meet the study criteria.

A conversion program survey questionnaire was designed to elicit information about the features of transition from a diploma to a degree-granting nursing education program. Open-ended questions were used to explore the following areas: program initiation and planning, initiation of arrangement, program approval and accreditation, program administration, institutional roles, curriculum, faculty and student responsibilities.

FINDINGS

Description of the Program

Twenty programs were located that had converted or were planning to convert to degree-granting status in 1982. All 20 programs were contacted and of these 17 agreed to participate in the study, a response rate of 85 percent. Of the 17, two programs were in the process of converting to baccalaureate programs and 15 programs had admitted students. Of the 15, eight programs awarded an associate degree in nursing, six programs awarded a baccalaureate degree in nursing and one program awarded a master's degree in nursing. Three of the programs continued to award a diploma along with a degree (see Table 1).

Table 1

Type of degree granted by number of respondents.

Associate degree	6
Associate degree plus diploma	2
Associate degree plus baccalaureate	1
Baccalaureate degree	4
Baccalaureate degree plus diploma	1
Master's degree	1
Programs in process of change to baccalaureate	2
TOTAL	17

Initiation and Planning

When asked to indicate the impetus for initiation of the program, respondents most frequently mentioned the desire to increase graduate mobility, national trends and increased need for an expanded knowledge base (see Table 2).

The median length of time between planning for and initiation of the new program was two years, with a range from one to nine years.

When asked to list the five major barriers encountered in the planning stage, respondents most frequently included credentialing, approval and major curriculum changes (see Table 3).

Table 2

Impetus for initiation of program by number of responses and percent of responses.

Impetus for Initiation of Program	Number of Responses*	Percent of Responses
National trends	10	(25.0)
Increased need for expanded knowledge base	8	(20.0)
Desire to increase graduate mobility	7	(18.0)
Decline in applicants for diploma program	3	(7.0)
Give students opportunity for collegiate atmosphere	2	(5.0)
State study recommendations	2	(5.0)
Desire to share college facilities/curricula	2	(5.0)
Cost of nursing school to hospital	2	(5.0)
Improved utilization of existing facilities	1	(2.5)
Increased availability of college/university education	1	(2.5)
Faculty commitment to baccalaureate education	1	(2.5)
Authorization of state board of regents	1	(2.5)
TOTAL	40	100

*Number of responses reflects multiple responses.

Initiation of Arrangement

Three models for conversion emerged from the survey: 1) schools of nursing that have made cooperative arrangements with universities to develop new degree-based programs; 2) schools of nursing that have closed their diploma programs and become independent degree-granting nursing schools; and 3) schools of nursing that have become part of large university programs and are utilizing their clinical resources for associate and/or baccalaureate education (see Table 4).

Coordination between Programs

Most of the program directors/deans (76 percent) indicated there is a designated liaison person between the school and cooperating agency. Job titles for this liaison varied from coordinator to coordinating committee (see Table 5).

Forty-one percent of the liaison persons reported to deans or directors of both the school of nursing and the affiliated university.

Program Approval/Accreditation

All respondents indicated having State Board of Nursing and State Board of Higher Education approval (or equivalent titles). Approximately 41 percent of all respondents indicated having National League for Nursing (NLN) accreditation. Respondents who did not have NLN accreditation indicated that they were seeking it.

Table 3

Major barrier encountered in the planning stage by category and by number and percent of responses.*

Barriers Encountered in the Planning Stage	Number of Responses	Percent of Responses**
Credentialing/Approval	20	(37.7)
■ Meeting criteria of state board of education	8	(15.0)
■ Meeting criteria of state board of nursing	6	(11.3)
■ Meeting criteria of National League for Nursing	4	(7.5)
■ Meeting criteria of regional association of universities and colleges	1	(1.8)
■ Confusion over hospital-based status	1	(1.8)
Faculty	9	(17.0)
■ Resistance to change	4	(7.5)
■ Unwilling to relinquish control	3	(5.6)
■ Need for re-education	2	(3.7)
Major Curriculum Changes	7	(13.0)
Administration	6	(11.0)
■ Change in organizational structures	4	(7.5)
■ Change in leadership during planning	1	(1.8)
■ Resistance from administrators from other hospitals	1	(1.8)
Resistance from Nursing Education Community	4	(7.5)
Establishment of Affiliations	3	(5.6)
Costs	3	(5.6)
Alumni Resistance	1	(1.8)
TOTAL	53	99.2

*Total percentage adds up to less than 100 percent due to error in rounding off.

**Number of responses reflects multiple responses.

Table 4

Type of arrangement between school of nursing and university by number of responses and percent response.

Type of Arrangement	Number of Responses	Percent Responses
Contract between school of nursing and university	10	(58)
Contract between schools of nursing and hospital for clinical facilities agreement	3	(18)
Agreement	3	(18)
Co-sponsorship with joint degree	1	(6)
TOTAL	17	(100)

Table 5

Job title by number of responses and percent response.

Job Title	Number of Responses	Percent Response*
Nursing education coordinator	5	29
Interinstitutional council	2	12
Coordinating committee	2	12
Coordinator of each specialty	1	6
Dean of nursing	1	6
Vice president, hospital and chairperson, division of nursing	1	6
President and academic dean	1	6
No title	3	18
Not applicable	1	6
TOTAL	17	101

*Total percentage greater than 100 due to rounding error.

Program Administration

Benefits

The university/college reported that improved recruitment of students, improved reputation and decreased costs by sharing facilities were major advantages resulting from the new program. The hospital/agency reported that improved recruitment of students and employees, improved reputation, improved level of patient care and decreased costs by sharing facilities were added advantages.

Institutional Roles

The proportion of program support provided by each institution in these cooperative arrangements varied. Seventeen percent of the directors/deans indicated there was an equal share arrangement between the universities and hospitals for program support. Thirty-eight percent indicated there were separate but equal financial arrangements. Forty-five percent of the directors/deans indicated that 95 percent of the program support was given by the hospital in the form of direct financing, staff time, services-in-kind, audio-visual equipment, dormitory space, classroom space and library resources.

Curriculum

New curricula were developed or were in the process of being developed by all of the conversion programs. The most common processes used were task force (32 percent), advisory committees (21 percent), consultants (17 percent) and faculty committees (10.5 percent). Joint ad hoc and planning committees were less commonly used (10.5 percent). Combinations of these methods were used nine percent of the time.

In the 10 programs with cooperative arrangements between universities and nursing schools, curriculum evaluation, revision, approval and implementation were conducted jointly (66.4 percent) but equally (33.6 percent). Independent, degree-granting schools of nursing retained full responsibilities for curricula.

Credit for transferred liberal arts and science courses and nursing courses was determined through challenge examination or previous course work (45 percent) and nursing courses (33 percent) (see Table 6).

Table 6

Method used to determine transfer of credit by type of course and percent of responses (for all programs).

	Type of Course		
Method Used to Determine Credit	**Liberal Arts**	**Science**	**Nursing**
Challenge exam	13.6	13.6	16.6
Credit for previous course work	27.2	27.2	22.2
Both methods	45.0	45.0	33.3
Not applicable	14.2	14.2	27.9

Program Curriculum

Students spent 50 percent of their time at the hospital/clinical site and 50 percent of their time at the college/university site. Academic credit was granted in similar proportions. Most of the programs offered course work only during the day.

A copy of the program curriculum plan was provided by most directors/deans (58 percent). Courses were grouped into categories of physical and biological sciences, social sciences, humanities, electives and nursing courses. The percentage of courses required for each category was calculated and the level of specificity and techniques for reporting hours varied between institutions; therefore, the percentages reported here are approximate. Nursing courses constituted approximately 41 percent of required course work in programs granting associate degrees. The cognate areas of physical and biological sciences, social sciences, humanities and electives constituted approximately 59 percent of required course work. The two programs granting both the diploma and associate degree required that approximately 35 percent of course work be completed in nursing and 65 percent in cognate areas.

Nursing courses constituted 41 percent of course work and cognate areas constituted 59 percent in programs granting baccalaureate degrees. These figures correspond very closely to figures reported by the National League for Nursing sample of baccalaureate programs (1979). Quiring and Gray reported that in 53 programs they surveyed, nursing courses constituted 43 percent of the total hours required for a degree and cognate area courses constituted 59 percent.

In the one program granting a diploma and a baccalaureate degree required that 68 percent of the total hours were in nursing courses and 32 percent in cognate area courses.

The one master's program courses and percentages varied with the level desired. The generalist level specified that 58 percent of total required hours be nursing courses and 42 percent be cognate area courses for graduation. The specialist level required 64 percent and 36 percent, respectively.

Faculty

Where cooperative arrangements existed between nursing schools and universities, faculty qualifications, selection, employment, salary, benefits, tenure and promotion were determined separately but equally. Sixty-five percent indicated that no changes were made in faculty. In the 14 percent of the programs where there were changes, 60 percent of the respondents indicated that faculty upgraded their credentials by obtaining higher degrees; 20 percent added directors for the new programs; and 20 percent received resignations from faculty members. The remaining 16 percent indicated that faculty changes had occurred as a result of natural attrition.

Faculty changes were also uncommon at the affiliated university. Eighty percent of the directors indicated that no university faculty changes were made. Of the 20 percent who indicated there were changes, half of the affiliated universities increased full-time faculty; one-quarter hired adjunct faculty to teach at the nursing school; and one-quarter offered master's-prepared hospital school of nursing faculty positions at the university.

In 76 percent of the nursing schools, new faculty employment arrangements occurred as a result of the new program. One-third of the respondents indicated that faculty had adjunct positions at the affiliated university; 4 percent indicated joint faculty appointments; 6.6 percent indicated faculty status had been upgraded from instructor levels; 6.6 percent had instituted new personnel policies; 6.6 percent had developed nursing consultation roles with the university; and 6.6 percent indicated they had some unemployment.

Students

Where cooperative arrangements existed between schools of nursing and universities, criteria for selection of students, receipt of tuition, determination of number of credits required for a degree, determination of source of academic and receipt of room and board payment were determined jointly 50 percent of the time and by the school of nursing 25 percent of the time (see Table 7).

Table 7

Determination of student factors by cooperating agencies and by number of responses and percent of responses.*

	School of Nursing		University		Both: Jointly		Both: Separately	
	(n)	(%)	(n)	(%)	(n)	(%)	(n)	(%)
Sets criteria of student selection	1	(16.6)	0	(0)	4	(66.4)	1	(16.6)
Selects students	0	(0)	0	(0)	5	(83)	1	(16.6)
Collects tuition	3	(50)	0	(0)	1	(16.6)	2	(33.2)
Determines number of credits required for degree	1	(16.6)	0	(0)	4	(66.4)	1	(16.6)
Determines sources of academic credits	1	(16.6)	1	(16.6)	3	(50)	1	(16.6)
Collects room and board	3	(50)	0	(0)	1	(16.6)	1	(16.6)
Average percent (rounded)		(25)		(2.7)		(50)		(19)

*Total percents are less than 100 due to rounding error.

Tuition per credit hour for both liberal arts courses and physical and biological science courses was equal to nursing courses 63 percent of the time (see Table 8).

Table 8

Comparison of tuition per credit hour by course type by percent response.

	Liberal Arts	**Physical/ Biological Sciences**	
Percent	19	25	Less than nursing courses
Response	13	12.5	More than nursing courses
	63	63	Equal to nursing courses

In this sample, the first class of students was graduated from the new program in 1974. In programs where graduations have already occurred, the average number of students graduated per year was 55, with a range from 4 to 87. Of the four respondents able to answer questions about graduates' employment status and location of graduates' employers, 82 percent of the graduates were employed at acute care hospitals within the state.

Ten respondents returned admission and eligibility policies required graduation from an accepted secondary school. Of these, 81 percent required SAT, ACT, CEEB scores; 54 percent required a grade of "C" or better in chemistry, biology and math; and 50 percent required graduation in the upper 50 percent of their class, letters of recommendation and interviews with the admissions committee or dean. One-third of the respondents required that the student have no health problems and two programs admitted only licensed practical nurses. The master's degree program required that applicants be non-nurse graduates with a bachelor of arts or sciences degree and have a grade point average of 3.0 or greater.

Various types of financial assistance were available for all 17 programs. Ninety-five percent of the respondents indicated the presence of state financial aid; 79 percent, federal aid; 76 percent, private scholarships; and 65 percent, hospital scholarships. Forty-one percent indicated that hospital and campus work-study programs were available and 35 percent indicated hospital tuition reimbursement as a source of financial aid. Twenty-three percent stated that loans were available and 6 percent indicated Veterans Administration benefits, Social Security and union-sponsored financial assistance were available. Combinations of these were also available.

Suggestions to Others

Of suggestions made to others considering the same type of program, program planning received the most comments (43.5 percent). Major suggestions were to provide enough planning time (15 percent), obtain consultation (15 percent), assess long-term needs for area (8.5 percent) and assess area colleges carefully (2 percent).

Suggestions regarding institutional roles had the next highest number of comments (12 percent). Suggestions regarding faculty (10.5 percent), students (9 percent), arrangement/agreement (8.5 percent), program administration (3.5 percent) and approval/accreditation (2 percent) were most prominent. "Have patience and a sense of humor" was also suggested (10 percent) (see Table 9).

Most of the respondents (73 percent) indicated they had used consultants in program planning; when specifically asked, almost all of the respondents (95 percent) recommended using consultants.

Table 9

Suggestions to others considering initiation of same type of program by number and percent of responses.*

	Number of Responses	Percent of Responses
Program Planning	25	(43.5)
Provide enough planning time	8	(15)
Obtain consultation	8	(13)
Assess long-term needs for area	5	(8.5)
Plan realistically	3	(5)
Assess area colleges carefully	1	(2)
Arrangement/Agreement	5	(8.5)
Make contract/agreement with university/college	5	(8.5)
Approval/Accreditation	1	(2)
Follow criteria for accrediting	1	(2)
Program Administration	2	(3.5)
Hire a coordinator early	2	(3.5)
Institutional Roles	7	(12)
Supportive hospital board of trustees	3	(5)
Supportive hospital administration	2	(3.5)
Have nursing school retain budgetary control	2	(3.5)
Faculty	6	(10.5)
Encourage faculty involvement	3	(5)
Have faculty decide on technical/professional issues	2	(3.5)
Have nursing school retain control of nursing faculty	1	(2)
Students	5	(9)
Identify competency for graduates	2	(3.5)
Encourage student involvement	2	(3.5)
Protect academic integrity of students	1	(2)
Other	6	(10)
Have patience and a sense of humor	6	(10)
TOTAL RESPONSES	58	(99)

*Total percent is less than 100 due to rounding error.

According to respondents, qualifications to look for in a consultant were knowledge of curriculum (77 percent), knowledge of credentialing (50 percent), open-mindedness and objectivity (38 percent) and knowledge of nursing education (33 percent).

IMPLICATIONS

Diploma nursing programs that have successfully made the transition to collegiate-based educational programs and that have maintained standards for accreditation are important models for nursing education and practice, as well as for other hospital/diploma schools contemplating a new direction. Methods found in this study that maintain use of existing educational resources, qualified faculty, libraries, classrooms and other resources will be useful to others.

References

Kintgen-Andrews, J. The development and demonstration of an articulation model. *Nursing and Health Care* 3:181, Apr. 1982.

National Commission on Nursing. *Summary of the Public Hearings.* Chicago: Hospital Research and Educational Trust, 1981.

National Commission on Nursing. *Initial Report and Preliminary Recommendations.* Chicago: Hospital Research and Educational Trust, 1981.

National Commission on Nursing. *Inventory of Innovative Programs and Projects.* Chicago: Hospital Research and Educational Trust, 1981.

Stevens, B.J. Program articulation: What it is and what it is not. *Nursing Outlook* 29:700, Dec. 1981.

Quiring, J.D. and Gray, G.T. Is baccalaureate education based on a patchwork curriculum? *Nursing Outlook* 27:708, Nov. 1979.

Ibid.

U.S. Department of Health and Human Services. *The Registered Nurse Population: An Overview from National Sample Survey of Registered Nurses, November 1980.* Report no. 82–5. Hyattsville, MD: U.S. Department of Health and Human Services, Division of Health Professions Analysis, June 1982.

Appendix 4

SURVEY OF SCHOOLS OF NURSING

The survey of schools of nursing was sent to all nursing schools accredited by the National League for Nursing: baccalaureate and higher degree (Bachelor of Science in Nursing), associate degree (Associate Degree in Nursing), diploma and practical (vocational) schools (Licensed Practical Nurse/Licensed Vocational Nurse). In this report of the survey, the term "nursing school" is used instead of nursing education program to allow differentiation of the school (or total program) from the more discrete programs such as mentor programs described.

Surveys were sent to schools of nursing in the United States. There are currently 283 Bachelor of Science in Nursing degree, 241 Diploma, 479 Associate Degree in Nursing and 751 Licensed Practical Nurse/Licensed Vocational Nurse degree National League for Nursing-accredited schools of nursing in the United States. Returns were received from 2,000 schools; of these, 1,754 were usable.

FINDINGS

More than one hospital was used for students' clinical experiences by most respondents. The total number of different hospitals used by reporting schools is shown in Table 1. Bachelor of Science in Nursing and higher degree schools reported use of more hospitals than did other types of schools: 29.3 percent of Bachelor of Science in Nursing and higher degree programs used more than 11 different hospitals compared with 8.8 percent of Associate Degree in Nursing schools, 1.3 percent of Licensed Practical Nurse/Licensed Vocational Nurse schools and 0.4 percent of diploma schools. The majority of all types of programs used from one to 10 hospitals.

Type of Arrangement

The type of administrative arrangements the school of nursing had with hospitals was examined. All types of nursing schools that responded to the survey indicated that contracts were most frequently used, followed by agreements and affiliations as shown in Table 2.

Table 1

Number of hospitals used by nursing schools for student clinical experience by type of school.

Type of Nursing School	Number of Hospitals				
	1–5	5–10	11–20	20+	Total
Bachelor of Science in Nursing and higher degree					
Percent	32.6	36.3	18.9	10.4	100
Number	(88)	(9.8)	(51)	(28)	(270)
Diploma					
Percent	87.8	9.2	0.4	0	
Number	(209)	(22)	(1)	0	(238)
Associate Degree in Nursing					
Percent	57.0	33.8	7.9	0.9	
Number	(268)	(159)	(37)	(4)	(470)
Licensed Practical Nurse					
Percent		86.8	9.3	1.3	—
Number	(653)	(70)	(10)	—	(752)
Total Percent	70.4	20.2	5.7	1.8	100
Total Number	(1218)	(349)	(99)	(32)	(1730)

Table 2

Type of arrangement by educational program.

	Bachelor of Science in Nursing		Diploma		Associate Degree in Nursing		Licensed Practical Nurse	
Arrangement	%	#	%	#	%	#	%	#
Contract	84.9	(241)	84.5	(202)	83.3	(400)	76.9	(572)
Affiliation	19.0	(54)	13.1	(91)	38.1	(63)	26.7	(199)
Agreement	55.6	(158)	45.0	(141)	59.0	(216)	45.0	(335)

When examined by region, schools with contracts and agreements were fairly evenly distributed: affiliations were reported most frequently by schools in the New England (30.6), Mid-Atlantic (30.0) and West South Central (27.4) regions. They were least frequent in the Mountain region.

Method of Contribution to Nursing Schools

The relationship between schools of nursing and hospitals can be partly explained by the type of contributions hospitals make to nursing education. Two categories of contributions were examined: financial and services and facilities. Table 3 shows the percentages of nursing schools receiving each type of contribution by type of school.

Table 3

Method of hospital contribution by type of nursing school.

	Type of Program							
	Bachelor of Science in Nursing		**Diploma**		**Associate Degree in Nursing**		**Licensed Practical Nurse**	
Method of Contribution	%	#	%	#	%	#	%	#
Financial								
Program Subsidy	4.2	(12)	20.7	(50)	4.4	(21)	8.1	(61)
Direct Financing	8.1	(23)	27.8	(67)	4.8	(23)	8.8	(66)
Services/Facilities								
Service in Kind	14.8	(42)	11.6	(28)	7.1	(34)	15.3	(115)
Staff Time	37.5	(106)	22	(53)	19.6	(94)	20.2	(152)
Space Allocation	48.4	(137)	42.3	(102)	37.6	(180)	37.5	(282)
Audio-Visual Equipment	20.5	(58)	23.2	(56)	17.3	(83)	24.9	(187)
Dormitory	8.4	(22)	45.4	(103)	21.8	(21)	4.9	(35)
Classroom	69.5	(182)	85	(193)	75.5	(330)	82.4	(587)
Library	88.5	(232)	91.2	(207)	81.5	(356)	85.1	(606)

Program subsidy was more frequent in the South Atlantic (20.2 percent), East North Central (19.6 percent) and West North Central (16.0 percent) regions; it was lowest in the Mountain (3.1) and Pacific (4.9) regions. All types of programs reported space allocation and use of audio-visual equipment at almost equal percentages. Regional variations in the other contributions are suggested. Services in kind were highest in the East and West North and West South Central regions, but lowest in the East South Central and Pacific regions. Staff time was highest in the East North Central, South Atlantic and Mid-Atlantic regions, but lowest in the East South Central, New England and Mountain regions.

Direct financing was reported by 9.9 percent of responding schools. Highest percentages of schools reporting direct financing were in the West South Central (17.7 percent), East North Central (15.1 percent) and West North Central (14.6 percent) regions. They were lowest in the Mountain (4.2 percent) and Pacific and East Central (7.3 percent, respectively) regions.

Contribution to Students

Hospitals also contribute to nursing schools through student support as indicated in Table 4. Opportunities for student employment were most frequently reported by all types of schools. Tuition reimbursement appears to be directed most frequently to Bachelor of Science in Nursing and higher degree programs. Scholarship programs are more frequent than loan programs for all types of schools.

Table 4

Type of hospital student financial support by type of nursing school.

	Bachelor of Science in Nursing		Diploma		Associate Degree in Nursing		Licensed Practical Nurse	
	%	#	%	#	%	#	%	#
Scholarship Program	25.4	(72)	19.5	(49)	31.3	(150)	20.5	(154)
Loan Program	7.4	(21)	15.4	(37)	11.1	(53)	8.3	(62)
Tuition Reimbursement	41.7	(118)	16.6	(40)	22.8	(109)	8.8	(66)
Opportunities for Student Employment	50.9	(137)	57.7	(131)	61.5	(270)	59.7	(390)

Faculty Involvement

Various types of faculty arrangements were reported by all types of programs. Table 5 shows the major types of arrangements reported by responding schools.

Table 5

Types of faculty arrangements with hospitals by type of school.

	Bachelor of Science in Nursing		Diploma		Associate Degree in Nursing		Licensed Practical Nurse	
Faculty Arrangement	%	#	%	#	%	#	%	#
Orientation for Faculty	95.9	(258)	95.6	(217)	90.2	(396)	80.9	(528)
Opportunities for Part-time Faculty Employment	88.3	(242)	78.7	(188)	86.1	(384)	64.3	(399)
Joint Faculty Appointments in Hospitals	33.2	(91)	10.5	(25)	5.2	(23)	4.3	(27)
Faculty Participation on Hospital Committees	64.2	(176)	96.2	(230)	43.3	(193)	46.5	(289)
Faculty Research in Hospitals	56.2	(144)	37.2	(89)	12.3	(5.5)	7.1	(44)
Nursing Staff Participation on Faculty Committees	52.2	(143)	62.8	(150)	44.6	(199)	58.3	(362)

Faculty participation on hospital committees appeared to be a feature of diploma schools, whereas joint faculty appointments and research were reported more frequently by Bachelor of Science in Nursing and higher degree programs. The presence of preceptor, mentor, internship and extern programs was examined by type of nursing school and by region of the country. Table 6 shows their location by type of school, and Table 7 gives information about the percentage of total nursing schools with preceptor, mentor, internship and extern schools and the breakdown of their location by region of the country.

There were more preceptor programs in the districts, territories and Mountain and Pacific states. The West North Central area had the greatest number of mentor programs, whereas intern programs were in greater numbers in the districts, territories and North East and East South Central regions. Extern programs were found in greater percentages in the East South Central region. The data suggest regional patterns for these programs and that different names may be used. In the West South Central region, for example, 6.9 percent of the schools had preceptor programs (average 11.1 percent); but 3.6 percent had mentor and 2.4 percent had internship programs (average 2.5 and 2.6, respectively).

Table 6

Provision of preceptor, mentor and internship programs by type of nursing school.

	Bachelor of Science in Nursing		Diploma		Associate Degree in Nursing		Licensed Practical Nurse	
	%	#	%	#	%	#	%	#
Preceptor	43.9	(118)	11.9	(27)	12.3	(54)	8.1	(53)
Mentor	15.2	(41)	5.7	(13)	5.9	(26)	7.8	(51)
Internship	11.2	(30)	4.0	(9)	10.7	(47)	3.8	(25)

Continuing Education

Schools of nursing and hospital arrangements for continuing education were explored. Cooperative planning was reported by more Bachelor of Science in Nursing and Associate Degree in Nursing programs than for other types. Less than 11 percent of all schools reported having contracts or agreements for continuing education (see Table 8).

Innovative Programs

Schools were asked to provide information about innovations. Table 9 gives information about the innovations reported. Articulation with another college or university was the most frequent innovation reported by Licensed Practical Nurse (37.5 percent), diploma (62.6 percent) and Associate Degree in Nursing (42.5 percent) schools. Preceptor, mentor or internship programs were the most frequent innovations for Bachelor of Science in Nursing and higher degree schools, followed by research.

Table 7

Regional distribution of preceptor, mentor and internship programs by percentage of schools with each and by total number of programs for each.

	Preceptor		**Mentor**		**Internship**		**Externship**	
	% of Schools	**% of Programs**	**% of Schools**	**% of Programs**	**% of Schools**	**% of Programs**	**% of Schools**	**% of Programs**
District/ Territory	19.0	1.9	–	–	4.8	2.0	–	–
North East	15.7	7.9	1.9	4.1	4.6	10.0	2.8	5.2
Mid-Atlantic	8.1	10.7	1.8	10.2	1.4	320.0	1.8	8.6
South Atlantic	11.7	18.1	1.8	12.2	4.2	28.0	3.9	22.4
East North Central	9.3	14.0	3.1	20.4	2.8	18.0	3.7	20.7
East South Central	13.5	8.4	0.8	2.0	3.8	10.0	8.3	19.0
West North Central	10.0	9.8	5.3	22.4	1.0	4.0	1.0	3.4
West South Central	6.9	7.9	3.6	18.4	2.4	12.0	2.8	12.1
Mountain	17.2	7.9	2.0	4.1	2.0	4.0	1.0	1.7
Pacific	16.1	13.5	1.7	6.1	1.1	4.0	2.2	6.9
Percentage	11.1	100	2.5	100	2.6	100	3.0	100

Table 8

Types of arrangements for continuing education by type of school.

	Bachelor of Science in Nursing		**Diploma**		**Associate Degree in Nursing**		**Licensed Practical Nurse**	
Continuing Education Arrangements	**%**	**#**	**%**	**#**	**%**	**#**	**%**	**#**
Contract	8.6	(23)	1.3	(3)	3.3	(15)	1.4	(10)
Agreement	10.9	(29)	3.0	(7)	9.1	(41)	4.1	(30)
Cooperative Planning	52.6	(140)	17.1	(40)	49.4	(224)	22.4	(162)

Table 9

Innovative programs by type of school.

Innovative Programs	Bachelor of Science in Nursing %	Bachelor of Science in Nursing #	Diploma %	Diploma #	Associate Degree in Nursing %	Associate Degree in Nursing #	Licensed Practical Nurse %	Licensed Practical Nurse #
Articulation with another college/university	26.9	63	42.5	137	62.6	107	37.5	142
Preceptor/internship/ mentor programs	54.3	127	21.4	69	11.7	20	7.1	27
Consortium for education, staff development or continuing education	33.8	79	38.5	124	22.8	39	32.7	124
Education methods: satellite/computer-assisted instruction	14.5	34	10.6	34	4.7	8	9.8	37
Work-study programs for students	26.1	61	25.8	83	29.2	50	22.2	84
Curriculum development	38.5	90	32.9	106	44.4	76	36.1	137
Research projects	47.0	110	9.0	29	14.6	25	5.0	19
Other	20.9	49	22.4	72	16.4	28	14.0	53

SUMMARY

Respondents were asked to comment on trends in the relationship between nursing education and nursing practice. Major themes reflected in the many comments were:

- finding new ways to collaborate,
- strengthening ties between education and practice,
- upgrading curriculum in schools, and
- upgrading qualifications of nurses in practice.

Among developing ways to incorporate contributions from nursing practice into nursing education and visa versa were: joint appointments; shared resources, particularly for continuing education; and committees for liaison planning and special projects. Of mutual benefit were programs for increasing the amount of clinical nursing research; involving qualified nurses in practice in the clinical education of nursing students; and having nurse faculty participate in nurse practice projects. Contracts with schools of nursing were being reviewed by nurse administrators to determine appropriate shared services or financial exchange of services. In general, the trends indicate strong efforts to improve and solidify relations between nursing education and nursing practice for the purpose of improving the quality of nursing care.

NATIONAL COMMISSION ON NURSING SURVEY OF NURSING EDUCATION IN HOSPITALS, 1982

This survey was conducted to explore administrative relationships and trends between hospitals and schools of nursing. The survey was sent to a random sample of 360 community hospitals, and 297 responses were received, an 82.5 percent return. Of the total, 241 operated a school of nursing. The type of nursing program, diploma or licensed practical nurse, was not indicated. Numbers of nurses employed varied from fewer than 100 to over 1000, with the majority of respondents having 200–500 nurses employed.

Hospitals were asked to indicate the number of schools of nursing with which they were associated and the types of arrangements they had with the schools. Table 1 shows the responses to this question.

Hospital Arrangements

Various types of arrangements were mentioned: 17.5 percent of the respondents had joint faculty appointments, 79.8 percent had faculty members on hospital nursing committees and 42.8 percent had hospital nurses on curriculum committees. A total of 60.6 percent (180) had full-time temporary employment for faculty and 30 percent (89) had research projects by or with faculty from schools of nursing. Hospital nurses served as mentors or preceptors for students in 54.2 percent (161) of responding hospitals.

Registered Nurse Staff Educational Preparation

Respondents were asked to give the highest level of educational preparation of registered nurses employed, as shown in Table 2.

Tuition Reimbursement

Of the responding hospitals, 93.9 percent indicated that they had tuition reimbursement programs for registered nurses. Table 3 shows the percentage of tuition reimbursed.

Table 1

Types of arrangements hospitals had with schools of nursing by type of nursing program.*

Type of Arrangement	Type of Nursing Program					
	(Percentages)					
	AD in Nursing	Diploma	BS in Nursing General	BS in Nursing Completion	MS in Nursing	Ph.D.
Contract	34.7	23.5	36.1	23.8	16.0	1.0
Affiliation	5.8	36.1	9.2	6.1	5.4	0.7
Agreement	15.0	19.7	15.0	16.0	14.6	1.0
Clinical Experience Only	33.0	27.6	36.1	23.5	16.7	0.7
Preceptor Program	2.4	5.1	9.5	8.8	9.5	0.3
Mentor Program	0.3	3.1	3.4	4.8	9.2	0.3
Internship Program	27.0	24.0	2.4	1.4	1.4	3.4
Student Employment	12.9	34.7	17.0	9.5	3.1	0.3
Continuing Education	4.4	9.2	6.8	6.1	3.7	0.7

*The random sample was one used by the American Hospital Association Data Center for Community Hospitals.

Table 2

Highest level of educational preparation for registered nurses employed in responding hospitals.

Range in Numbers	Associate Degree in Nursing		Diploma		Bachelor of Science in Nursing		Master of Science in Nursing		Doctorate	
	#	%	#	%	#	%	#	%	#	%
0–0	15	6.0	1	0.4	3	1.2	76	30.5	244	81.8
1–10	95	38.2	3	1.2	94	37.8	171	68.7	5	2.0
11–20	77	30.9	4	1.6	84	33.7	2	0.8		
21–30	46	18.5	7	2.8	52	20.9				
31–40	9	3.6	15	6.0	6	2.0				
41–50	3	1.2	28	11.2	10	3.4				
51–60	2	0.8	46	18.5						
61–70	—	—	53	21.3						
71–80	2	0.8	46	18.5						
81–90	—	—	35	14.1						
91–100	—	—	11	4.4						

Table 3

Percentage of tuition reimbursed by hospitals for registered nurse students.

Percentage of Tuition Reimbursed	Hospitals	
	#	%
1–25 percent	10	3.4
26–50 percent	42	14.1
51–75 percent	55	18.5
76–100 percent	139	46.8
No Answer	51	17.2
Total	297	100

Expectations of Faculty

The majority of responding hospitals (90.6 percent, or 269) required orientation for faculty, and 39.7 percent (118) required faculty to demonstrate clinical competence. Methods used to demonstrate clinical competence included curriculum vitae (32.2 percent), demonstrated practice in hospital (27.2 percent) and testing (6.2 percent). Also mentioned were validation from school, written references and experience records.

Orientation of New Graduates

A total of 99.3 percent (295) of respondents had an orientation program for new graduates. Of this number, 54.2 percent indicated that the program was standard for all new employees, while 46.1 percent reported having a self-paced orientation program. Table 4 shows the range of time for orientation programs of all types reported, and Table 5 gives the range of time for individualized programs.

Respondents were asked whether they thought newly graduated nurses were prepared for practice: 14.9 percent indicated "infrequently," 32.9 percent indicated "sometimes," 50.5 percent indicated "usually," 1.7 indicated "always," and 2.7 percent did not respond.

Table 4

Length of time in months for orientation program for new graduates by percentage of responding hospitals.

Length of Time in Months	Respondents	
	#	%
Up to 1	63	21.2
1–2	46	15.5
2–3	16	5.4
3–4	2	0.7
6	29	9.8
Length does not apply	133	44.8

Table 5

Range of weeks for individualized orientation programs for new graduate registered nurses.

Number of Weeks	Minimum Range		Maximum Range	
	#	%	#	%
1–2	72	24.2	75	25.2
3–4	95	32.0	83	2.0
5–6	21	7.1	46	14.8
7–8	9	6.8	2	0.7
10–12	5	2.7	9	2.0

Clinical Advancement Programs/Mode of Nursing Care Delivery

Clinical advancement programs were reported by 27.8 percent (81) of the respondents. The majority (46.3 percent, or 124) indicated that they used team nursing, 21.6 percent (58) indicated that they used modular nursing and 14.2 (38) indicated that they used primary nursing as the major mode of nursing care. The remainder either did not answer the question (10.1 percent) or indicated that they used combinations of the above.

Certification for Practice

Certification tests prior to employment were required by 15.5 percent of respondents, and 30.3 percent indicated that the certification tests were required for intensive care unit employment. Another 18 percent indicated that certification was required in special care areas including the operating room, emergency room and neonatal intensive care units.

Clinical Specialists/Nurse Practitioners

Over three-fourths of the respondents (76.2 percent, or 224) indicated that they employed nurse specialists. Of respondents with nurses having the title "clinical specialist," 44.7 percent (132) had from one to five such nurses and 10 percent (30) had from six to 10. Only 2.6 percent (9) of respondents had more than 10 clinical specialists.

Other categories of nurse specialists employed included nurse practitioners (79), nurse midwives (24) and nurse anesthetists (121).

Refresher Course for Registered Nurses

Refresher courses for registered nurses were offered by 28.6 percent (85) of the respondents.

Staff Development Departments

Staff development departments were reported by 98 percent (291) of the respondents. The majority of these (68.7 percent) were located in the department of nursing, and 28.6 percent were located in a centralized education department. Numbers of instructors employed by staff development departments are shown in Table 6.

Table 6

Number of instructors employed by staff development departments in responding hospitals.

Number of Instructors	Responding Hospitals	
	#	%
1–5	179	60.2
6–10	77	25.9
11–15	26	8.7
16–30	6	1.8

Cooperative Continuing Education

A number of resources were reported for continuing education for registered nurses. Of the respondents, 40 percent offered continuing education (118) with another college or university, 14.1 percent (42) with a junior college and 39 percent (112) with another hospital. Of the total, 91.9 percent had a nursing library (273) and 46.8 percent had a learning resource center (139).

Resources Provided by Hospitals for Schools of Nursing

The survey further explored relationships between hospitals and schools of nursing by asking the types of resources the hospital provided for educational programs. Table 7 shows the types of support.

Table 7

Types of support hospitals provide for schools of nursing by percentage of hospitals offering the support.

Type of Support	Percentages Offering Support by Type	
	#	%
Finance Operations of School	239	80.5
Classrooms/Lockers	228	76.8
Facilities/Dormitory	195	65.7
Faculty Wage Subsidy	191	64.3
Shared Services	177	59.6
Scholarship Program	141	47.5
Student Loans	139	47.1
Direct Payment to Student	92	31.2
Work-Study Programs	90	30.3

Effectiveness of Hospital-School Relationships

Respondents were asked about their relationships with schools of nursing: 72.9 percent indicated that they were highly effective; 25.1 percent, somewhat effective; 1.7 percent, slightly effective; and 0.3 percent, not at all effective.

Benefit of School to Hospital

Relationships with schools of nursing were said to be beneficial to the hospital as a source of recruitment of new graduates (98.6 percent), to stimulate nursing staff (92.3 percent) and to improve the quality of patient care given by the nursing department (83.0 percent).

Trends in the Hospital-School Relationship

Comments made in response to the query about anticipated changes and trends in the nursing education and hospital nursing service relationship included a wide variety of topics. Predominant was the trend to upgrade nursing education and to increase hospital alliances with schools of nursing.

General

Factors cited to result in improved relationships of hospitals with schools of nursing were strong internship programs, centralized education departments, the growth of baccalaureate completion programs and master's and doctoral programs in nursing, the designation of hospitals as a clinical resource for schools of nursing in colleges and universities and increased need for career mobility options for registered nurses.

Acceleration of the improved relationships between schools of nursing and hospitals were cited to result from increased specialization in nursing care, need for increased clinical knowledge and experience, development of research in nursing practice and the benefit of shared services with schools that helped both the nursing service in hospitals and schools of nursing. Several respondents commented that they were soliciting affiliations with colleges and universities to improve their community visibility and to improve retention of registered nurses at the hospital. An aggressive, collaborative approach to bringing nursing education and practice together was cited to improve consumers' trust in the hospital related to their safety and welfare and to help nurses and others reach a common understanding about expectations of nurse graduates and about current nursing practice. Respondents indicated that improved dialogue between the hospital and college was stated to lead to better planning and management of clinical experiences, shared funding for continuing education and other needed developmental projects.

The growing interdependence between education and service was related by many respondents to increased emphasis on clinical excellence and fiscal pressures. Evidence given by respondents of this interdependence included: increased requests to hospitals for preceptors for graduate nursing students, development of career ladders, increased use of educational technology and shared planning. Several respondents commented that broader involvement of hospitals with schools of nursing on college and university campuses resulted in improved nurse-physician and multidisciplinary relationships, as well as expanded resources for planning and development that were stimulated by cooperative effort. In several settings, continuing education had been extended to all nurses in the community, including those in physicians' offices and other settings.

Increased numbers of master's and doctoral level programs were thought to have stimulated improved resource sharing and communications and an increase in research. Table 8 shows the types of arrangements mentioned.

Comments from Hospital-based RN Schools

Many of the survey comments related to transition in nursing education. About 15 respondents indicated that they expected no change in their diploma programs. A few respondents said that they would strengthen and expand their programs. Three

Table 8

Types of arrangements between hospitals and schools of nursing.

Arrangements	Percentage of Hospitals	
	#	%
Internship, Preceptor, and Mentor Programs	155	52.5
Educational Consortium: Staff Development	108	36.4
Research Projects	78	26.3
Satellite Programs: Educational Technology	23	7.7

indicated that they were being forced to seek an alternative to the diploma program, seven indicated that they were exploring a move to baccalaureate education and 16 indicated that their schools were closing, often with arrangements for a new baccalaureate program. Educational mobility was commented on by 33 respondents who had plans under way to develop articulated educational programs.

Reasons given for closing diploma schools of nursing were: increased competition for students, cost of the school to the hospital, low retention rate of diploma school graduates in employment, ability to effectively recruit graduates from other nursing school programs, increased flexibility and cooperation of college-based programs in the area to supply adequate numbers of graduates, the benefits of reciprocal appointments (clinical and adjunct faculty), increased need to recruit baccalaureate and master's-prepared nurses in the hospital setting and the benefit of shared task force effort to develop change in nursing service and education.

Other less frequently cited reasons were increased competition among schools for clinical experiences for student nurses and the need to upgrade registered nurse qualifications to deal with increased acuity of patient need and the growth of ambulatory care services.

Glossary

This glossary of terms was developed by the commission throughout its deliberations and applies not only to the *Summary Report and Recommendations,* but to the *Initial Report and Preliminary Recommendations* and other commission publications. The glossary is arranged in nine categories:

- career;
- credentialing;
- general;
- management;
- nursing education;
- practice settings;
- standards of nursing practice;
- type of nursing education programs; and
- types of nursing positions.

The terms within each category are arranged alphabetically.

CATEGORY: CAREER

Career Ladder

Refers to a health care agency's system for promotion of nurses to recognize and reward individuals for education, experience, and performance in nursing practice. Levels of the career ladder are staged in incrementally more comprehensive roles and functions and may be differentiated by administrative, educational, or clinical practice functions.

Career Opportunities

In nursing, the types of positions in various practice settings that are available to qualified nurses. Some positions have specified experience or educational requisites. A nurse may seek a career path within an institution through a career ladder program or may move from one type of position to another within an institution or in different practice settings.

Career Pattern

The educational and employment experience a person selects in development of a personal career based on personal motivation and competence and available opportunities.

Educational Mobility

Educational plans that facilitate articulation of completed educational segments with additional learning in such a way that a student is able to work toward a higher credential in the same field without undue repetition.

CATEGORY: CREDENTIALING

Accreditation

A voluntary process of peer evaluation by which institutions and/or programs are appraised in relation to predetermined criteria and are publically recognized if there is compliance.

Certification

The process by which a nongovernmental agency or association attests that an individual has met certain predetermined standards specified by the certifying body to assure the public that the individual has mastered a body of knowledge and acquired skills in a particular specialty.

Credentialing

A broad term encompassing those processes that determine an individual's institution's and/or program's compliance with established standards.

Licensure

A process by which state government ensures a minimum level of competence and grants legal permission to individuals and agencies to engage in a designated practice or to provide a specific service.

Registration

A process by which qualified individuals are listed on an official roster maintained by a governmental or nongovernmental agency.

CATEGORY: GENERAL

Clinical Decision Making

Decisions made about patient care. In nursing, refers to decisions about patient needs for physical, social, and psychological care; patient teaching; counseling; and referral for continuity of care.

Competence

The quality of exercising judgment; possession of the required skill, knowledge, qualification, or capacity. Competence: having suitable or sufficient knowledge and skill.

Nurse-Physician Collaboration

A jointly determined relationship between the nurses and physicians working together in practice. The purpose of the collaboration is to integrate their care regimens into a single comprehensive approach to their patients' needs. The practitioners themselves define their roles in consonance with state laws, professional practice acts, policies of the hospital, and the special clinical needs of their particular practice field.

Nursing Shortage

The situation where employers of nurses in a given area cannot find the numbers and/or types of nurses they seek to employ for specific functions and shifts for the salaries, fringe benefits, and working conditions they are prepared to offer.

Supplementary Agency

An agency that employs, assigns, and pays nurses to work on a temporary basis in hospitals contracting with that agency.

Turnover

The turnover rate for a particular group of workers can be calculated by using the following formula:

$$\text{Annual Turnover Rate} = \frac{\text{Number of terminations per year}}{\text{Average number of employees for the unit}} \times 100$$

Vacant Budgeted Positions

Those budgeted positions which are currently unfilled or vacant of qualified personnel for which the hospital is actively seeking either a full-time or part-time replacement.

CATEGORY: MANAGEMENT

Ancillary Services

Those professional services other than medical and nursing services, such as laboratory, radiology, pharmacy, and therapy services that are provided to hospital patients in the course of care.

Decentralized (ization)

The implementation of a high degree of delegation of duties, power, and authority to lower levels of an organization.

Department

A distinct area or branch of an enterprise over which a manager has authority for the performance of specified activities.

Division

An administrative unit of an organization, bureau, or agency.

Hospital Department Groups

Patient Care Units (also called Nursing Units)	Medical and Surgical Units, Pediatric Units, Psychiatric Units, Obstetric Units, Newborn Nursery, Intensive Care Units, Non-Acute Units, Critical Care Units.
Diagnostic Services	Diagnostic Radiology, Electrodiagnosis, Nuclear Medicine, and Laboratory.
Operative Services	Anesthesiology, Ambulatory Surgery, Operating Room, Recovery Room, Delivery Room, Minor Surgery Room.

Therapeutic Services	Hemodialysis, Respiratory Therapy, Pharmacy, Intraveneous Therapy, Occupational Therapy, Pastoral Care, and Social Services.
Outpatient Services	Emergency Room, Clinic, Ambulatory Clinical Service, Oncology, Rehabilitation.
Support Service	Transportation, Central Services, Dietary, Housekeeping, In-House Laundry, Contract Laundry.
Other Professional Services	Medical Records, Education, Medical Care Evaluation.
Administrative Services	Nursing Administration, Fiscal Services, Security Data Processing, Administrative Services, other operating and non-operating services, Human Resources (Personnel).

Hospital Information System

Administrative and patient care data combined into a common set of data files for computer processing. These systems have the potential to increase efficiency through consolidation, coordination, and communication of massive quantities of data.

Management Unit

An organizational unit with its own hierarchy and subdivisions of responsibilities.

Participative Management

The style of management in which the leader encourages members of an organization to contribute ideas, opinions, and recommendations. Communication travels in an upward, as well as downward, manner and group decision making is promoted.

CATEGORY: NURSING EDUCATION

Articulated Educational Programs

A sequence of academic advancement planned between programs to increase educational and career mobility without duplication of previous learning experience.

Continuing Education

Planned, organized learning experiences designed to augment the knowledge, skills, and attitudes of registered nurses for the enhancement of nursing practice, education, administration, and research, to the end of improving health care to the public.

Externship

A program for nursing students, which includes clinical experiences in a variety of settings to improve student adjustment to the practice setting of nursing.

Internship

A program for graduate nurses to improve clinical proficiency and adjustment to the role of staff nurse.

Mentor

A person higher up on the organizational ladder, an authority in his or her field, a person of influence who commits time and emotion to a relationship with a less-experienced employee and is interested in the "mentoree's" personal growth and development; someone who boosts the mentoree's self-esteem and offers counsel and advice, and gives upward mobility to the mentoree's career.

Nontraditional Education

Common features of nontraditional nursing education are: 1) granting advanced placement for prior education or experience through challenge examinations or equivalency; 2) multiple exit and re-entry program designs; 3) programs designed for registered nurses only; 4) use of self-paced learning methods; 5) independent study programs; and 6) flexible schedules such as weekends or evenings.

Orientation

A program of learning experiences designed to prepare a graduate nurse to function within the unique environment of a specific institution. Such a program does *not* attempt to provide a continuation of basic nursing education but rather focuses on instruction designed to facilitate any necessary application of previously learned knowledge and skills to the requirements of the particular work situation. The duration of an orientation program is three months or less.

Preceptor

An experienced professional who is responsible for teaching and direct supervision of a student in the same profession who is undertaking professional responsibilities and duties.

Re-Entry/Refresher Course

A program to provide nurses who have not had recent clinical experience with a review of the theoretical basis of nursing, an introduction to new concepts in nursing, and an update of clinical skills.

Staff Development

A term describing a process that includes both formal and informal learning opportunities to assist individuals to perform competently in fulfillment of role expectations within a specific agency. Resources both within and outside the agency are utilized to facilitate the process.

CATEGORY: PRACTICE SETTINGS

Community Hospitals

All non federal, short-term, general and other special hospitals excluding hospital units of institutions whose facilities and services are available to the public.

Federal Government Health Care Agency

A health care agency that is managed by an agency or department of federal government.

Long-Term Care

A health care agency in which the average length of stay is 30 days or more or in which more than 50 percent of all patients are admitted to units where the average length of stay is 30 days or more.

Nonfederal Government Health Care Agency

A health care agency that is managed by an agency or department of state or local government.

Nongovernmental, Not-For-Profit Health Care Agency

A health care agency that operates on a not-for-profit basis under the ownership and control of a private corporation.

Proprietary (Also Known as For-Profit or Investor-Owned)

A health care agency that is owned and operated by a corporation or an individual and that operates on a for-profit basis.

Rural Hospital

An acute care hospital located outside a standard metropolitan statistical area.

Short-Term Care

A health care agency in which the average length of stay is less than 30 days or in which 50 percent of all patients are admitted to units where the average length of stay is less than 30 days.

Small Hospital

A hospital that has less than 100 acute care beds or has 4000 or less admissions per year.

CATEGORY: STANDARDS OF NURSING PRACTICE

Standards of Nursing Practice

Criteria set by the profession about the structure, process, and outcome of nursing practice against which quantitative or qualitative data can be evaluated.

CATEGORY: TYPE OF NURSING EDUCATION PROGRAM

The terms in this section are sequentially arranged by time and program, rather than alphabetically. Please note that degree titles at the bachelor's level and above depend on individual institutional policy.

Associate Degree in Nursing

Basic nursing education generally provided in a two-year community college that leads to an associate degree in nursing.

Diploma in Nursing

Basic nursing education provided in a two- or three-year hospital-based program that leads to a diploma in nursing.

Baccalaureate in Nursing

Basic nursing education provided through a four-year college or university that leads to a bachelor's degree with a major in nursing.

Master's in Nursing

A graduate degree program in nursing in which students acquire advanced knowledge from the biological and social sciences and develop competency in selected specialized clinical areas (such as gerontology, pediatrics, or psychiatric nursing) and functional areas (such as nursing education, research, administration, or clinical nursing.)

Doctorate in Nursing

The focus or purpose of doctoral education in nursing may be on clinical competence, theory development and research, preparation for a functional role, or any combination of these. One school offers the doctorate in nursing as the first professional degree. The title of the degree awarded depends on individual institutional policy and the purpose of the program.

CATEGORY: TYPES OF NURSING POSITIONS

Assisting Personnel

Personnel who function under the direct supervision of a registered nurse.

Community Health Nursing/Public Health Nursing

Refers to the application of prevention, health promotion, and maintenance services to populations of individuals and groups within their own environment of home, school, clinic, or work place in the community and the application of public health measures to the community as a whole. Public health nurses often function on multidisciplinary teams in developing and implementing health programs.

Nurse Administrator

Registered nurse accountable for nursing practice and for overall administration and management of nursing services provided in a health care agency.

Nurse Generalist

Registered nurses, graduated from an associate degree, diploma, or baccalaureate nursing program, who provide patient care in hospitals and nursing homes. The baccalaureate degree prepares the registered nurse to function in community nursing services, health agencies, schools, and industry.

Nurse Specialist

Registered nurse graduated from a master's in nursing program or a doctoral program who provides leadership; functions in education, administration, clinical specialty, or research; and is eligible for certification through a professional society.

Specialty

Specialty areas can be defined along three separate dimensions:

- health care needs (alcoholic, burn, cardiovascular, diabetic);
- population characteristics (infant, child, adolescent, adult, aged, family, community); and
- settings (community, hospital, industry, nursing home, school).

ORDER FORM

To: The Hospital Research and Educational Trust
840 North Lake Shore Drive
Chicago, Illinois 60611

No. of Copies	
	Source Book (#654300) 139 pages. $12.00 per copy.
	Summary Report and Recommendations (#654200) 43 pages. $7.00 per copy. A 10-percent discount applies on all orders of 10 or more copies.
	Nursing in Transition: Models for Successful Organizational Change (#654650) 53 pages. $7.00 per copy.
	Report of the Survey of Innovative Programs and Projects (#654640) 129 pages. $8.50 per copy.
	Initial Report and Preliminary Recommendations (#643100) 80 pages. $7.50 per copy. A 25-percent discount applies on all orders of 10 or more copies.
	Summary of the Public Hearings (#643635) 77 pages. $7.50 per copy. A 25-percent discount applies on all orders of 10 or more copies.
$	**Amount Enclosed**

Billed Orders

Purchase order no.

Name

Title/Division

Organization

Address

Billed orders must be written on a company purchase order with the name and phone number of a person to contact for confirmation. Minimum billed order: $25.00. Orders that are fully prepaid are not charged for shipping and handling. Billed orders are charged for shipping based on actual shipping costs. Sales tax must be paid on orders shipped to Illinois. If exempt, show exemption number: ___________

Please make all checks payable to:
The Hospital Research and Educational Trust.